A NEW HISTORY OF CATARACT SURGERY

PART 4

THE BRITISH ISLES BEFORE 1800

edited by

Christopher T. Leffler

This is the standard softcover print-on-demand edition—an accessible and budget-friendly version of this work. For those who appreciate quality, a premium hardcover edition with high-quality color illustrations is also available. Visit our website for more information.

ISBN: 978-90-6299-479-3

Wayenborgh Publishing
P.O. Box 20538
1001 NM Amsterdam, The Netherlands
www.historyophthalmology.com

Wayenborgh Publishing is an imprint of Kugler Publications, P.O. 20538, 1001 NM, Amsterdam, The Netherlands

Table of Contents

1. Early Cataract Surgery in the British Isles (Antiquity to 1800)

Christopher T. Leffler, MD, MPH[1]
Stephen G. Schwartz, MD, MBA[2]

Introduction

Cataract surgery may have been performed in the British Isles during antiquity in the form of couching, which involves displacing a cataract into the vitreous and out of the visual axis. Much of the history of this procedure in the British Isles from antiquity through the medieval and early modern periods has been poorly understood because early records are sparse and because historians have tended to assume that whatever was happening in antiquity must have been happening in the medieval period, or that what happened in Italy must have been happening in the British Isles also. Recent scholarship has looked in greater detail at the ophthalmic history in this region.[3]

If cataract couching was performed in Roman Britain, then it probably experienced the same decline during the "Dark Ages" that was seen in Latin-speaking Western Europe. Many historians have assumed that cataract couching was present in the British Isles throughout the medieval period. However, there is no solid evidence of cataract surgery in that region until the Elizabethan era (1558-1603), at which point there is ample documentation of many practitioners performing the procedure and of patients having it performed.

Roman Britain (43-410 CE)

In the time of the Caesars, there was a Celtic eye surgeon in Britain named Ariovist. Galen mentioned the eye salve of a British oculist named Stolus. Archaeologists have identified at least nine Roman instruments from seven sites, which might be cataract needles. However, seven of the nine instruments have the tip or the entire needle broken off, leaving some doubt about the original structure. Moreover, even when a complete instrument has been found, the original purpose cannot be

---

1 Department of Ophthalmology, Virginia Commonwealth University, Richmond, VA USA.

2 Department of Ophthalmology, Bascom Palmer Eye Institute, University of Miami Miller School of Medicine, Naples, FL, USA. Partially funded by NIH Center Core Grant P30EY014801 and by an Unrestricted Grant from Research to Prevent Blindness to the University of Miami.

3 Leffler et al. "Elizabethan" 2014; Leffler et al. "Stepkins" 2014; Leffler & Schwartz "Woolhouse" 2017; Leffler et al. "British Isles" 2021.

known with certainty. Roman surgical needles had a variety of uses besides cataract surgery: fine dissection, puncturing abscesses or hemorrhoids, raising the eyelid skin, transfixing small conjunctival masses, probing, or cautery. At least three of the instruments from one site were made of iron, three instruments were made of copper alloy, and one isolated handle was made of bone. One find has been dated to the 1st century, and one from the 2nd century, but the majority could date from any century of the Roman occupation (43-410).[4]

Absence of Medieval Records of Cataract Couching (410-1500)

Until recently, it has often been assumed that if cataract couching took place anywhere in medieval Europe, then it must have been present quite broadly, including in the British Isles.[5] However, we have been unable to identify in medieval Britain a single doctor who performed cataract couching, any witnesses to the procedure, or any patients who were considered for the procedure.

One could argue that the absence of specific names of doctors, witnesses, or patients stems from a paucity of records. However, from Andalusia to Japan, and from Cairo to Tournai, firsthand reports of medieval cataract couching have survived.

Moreover, several sources provide detailed information about medieval medicine in the British Isles. Some procedures were probably quite common in the medieval British Isles: bloodletting, cautery, scarification, lancing abscesses, drawing teeth, treatment of wounds and burns, and setting fractured bones. Other procedures were less common but were performed when indicated, including amputation, removal of arrows, and suturing of skin or intestinal injuries. Finally, some surgeries were performed by the occasional practitioners: lithotomy, hernia, and fistula-in-ano.[6]

High Middle Ages (c. 1066-1272) in England

The Norman invasion led by William the Conqueror of 1066 could have exposed the English to medicine from Continental Europe and the Mediterranean. The Normans were not only based in France but also held Sicily, Naples, and Antioch, beginning in the 11th century. Nonetheless, there is no solid evidence that these links did actually result in cataract couching in medieval England. A roster of British physicians from 500 to 1154 lists no oculists. Bishop William Warelwast of Exeter, of

---

4 Leffler et al. "British Isles" 2021.

5 Leffler et al. "British Isles" 2021.

6 Leffler et al. "British Isles" 2021.

the early 12th century, was pilloried for continuing to serve despite poor eyesight but was not noted to have had his vision restored surgically.[7]

Other types of ophthalmic care are recorded in England in this period. Roger of Lacock, the royal physician (d. 1233), made an eye ointment with fennel, rue, musk, and attic honey. Baldwin, a physician and abbot of St. Edmundsbury (d. 1097), traveled to Rome in 1071 to appeal a political dispute with a bishop named Arfast to the pope. Arfast subsequently suffered an eye injury from a thorn while riding through the forest. Baldwin only agreed to treat Arfast's eye after receiving written guarantees that Arfast would not pursue their political dispute.[8]

Historians have sometimes attributed miraculous cures of blindness during the medieval period to cataract couching. Such miraculous cures do survive in the biographical literature. Hamelin de Warenne, Earl of Surrey (c. 1130–1202), was said to be cured of his blindness from an "albugo" (white spot) in one eye by touching a covering from the tomb of Thomas Becket, who was murdered in 1170. This cure was viewed as a miracle, which justified Becket's sainthood. However, not all of Warenne's treatment required a miracle. Master Henry Grossus, a physician, made an eye lotion for the Earl Warenne. Moreover, Warenne held not only a castle in Yorkshire but also castles in Normandy, and he traveled in 1176 through central and southern France to attend his niece's wedding in Sicily. Thus, even if Hamelin's seemingly miraculous cure in one eye was really the result of a cataract surgery, the surgery might have taken place in France or Italy. Incidentally, St. Thomas' Hospital, the site of the first intraocular lens implantation in the modern era, received its name from Thomas Becket, the ophthalmic miracle worker.[9]

To the extent that clergy in the British Isles might have performed cataract couching during the early Middle Ages, such activities would have seen a decline after a series of religious edicts limiting or forbidding the study or practice of medicine by the clergy, including that of the Council of Tours in 1163. Such regulations might not have been enforced absolutely in all areas, but there does seem to be a dramatic decline in monastic medical activities by the end of the 1200s.[10]

Likewise, some of the early medieval oculists, such as Rabbi Abiatar Aben-Crexcas, and possibly Benevenutus Grassus, came from Jewish families. It is conceivable that the expulsion of Jews from England in 1290 was another event that reduced medical and surgical knowledge in the region.[11]

The word "cataract" evidently made its way into Norman French manuscripts in medieval Britain. The *Practica Brevis of Platearius* might have been written by

---

7 Leffler et al. "British Isles" 2021.

8 Leffler et al. "British Isles" 2021.

9 Leffler et al. "British Isles" 2021.

10 Leffler et al. "British Isles" 2021.

11 Leffler et al. "British Isles" 2021.

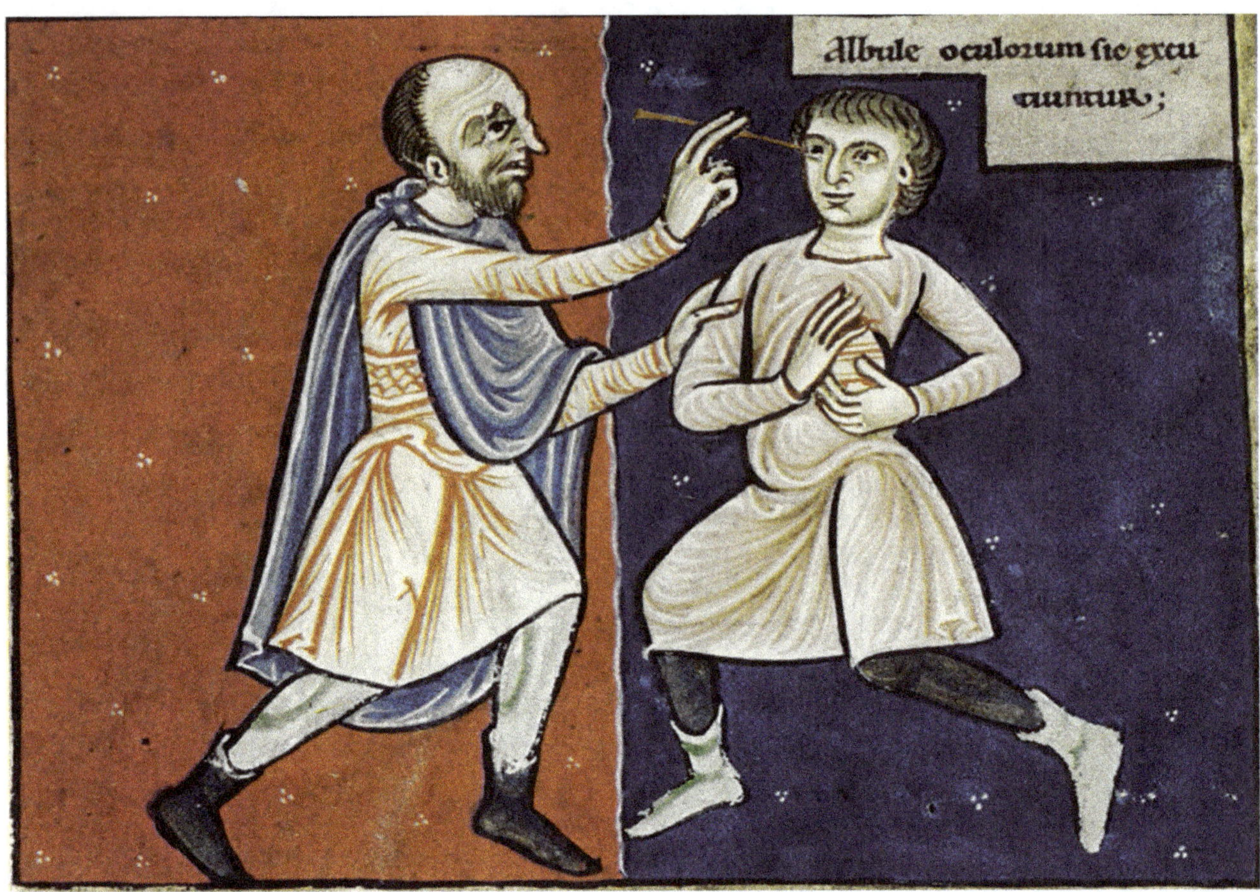

Fig. 1. A manuscript from England from the end of the 12th century (Ashmole 1462) contains the text: *"Albulae oculorum sic excutiuntur"*

Johannes Platearius II, of Salerno, Italy, between 1120 and 1150. A translation into Anglo-Norman (French) of this manuscript has a book *De egritudinibus oculorum* (*Of Eye Disease*), which notes: "Les ca[ta]ractes des eus sont a la fiez curable, a la fiez nient curable. Les curables garist l'en de .i. estrument de cyrugie, c'est asavoir de .i. aguille."[12] The Practica Brevis was also translated into Middle English. Therefore, at least a superficial awareness of cataract surgery circulated in Norman Britain.

Illustrations have played a role in the thinking of some historians. A manuscript from England from the end of the 12th century (Ashmole 1462) contains the text: *Albulae oculorum sic excutiuntur*, with a patient standing while an eye doctor approaches his eye with a rod (Fig.1).[13] A similar color figure and text are found in MS Sloane 1975, dating from the last quarter of the 12th century in either England

---

12 Leffler et al. "British Isles" 2021.

13 No author listed, Ashmole 1462 (folio 10) held at the Bodleian Library, Oxford (Leffler et al. "British Isles" 2021).

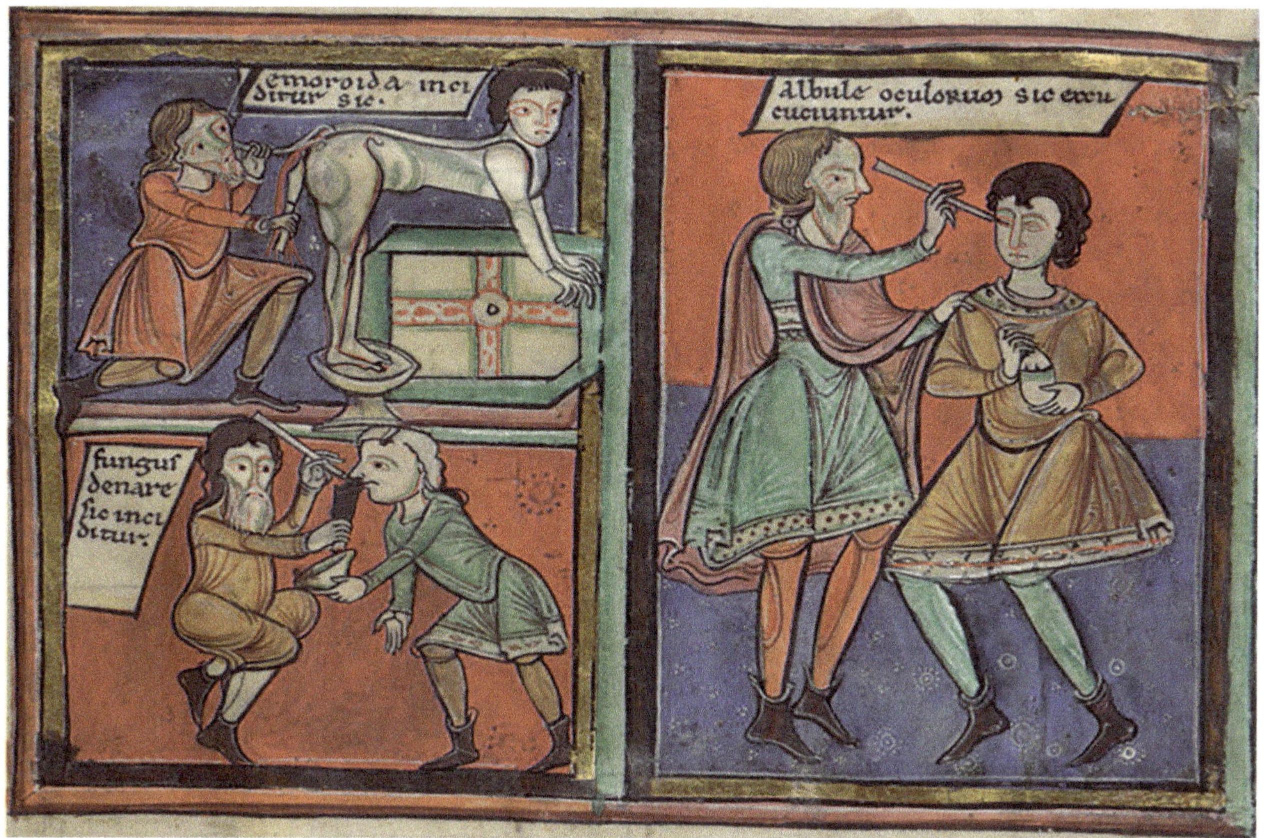

Fig. 2. Manuscript Sloane 1975, dating from the last quarter of the 12th century in either England or France.

or France (Fig.2).[14] Finally, a similar figure and text are found in Harley 1585, a manuscript of the third quarter of the 12th century, from either the Mosan region of the Netherlands or England (Fig. 3).[15] However, *albule oculorum* simply refers to a white spot on the eye, and there is no way to know if this spot is due to a pterygium, scarring from smallpox or keratitis, or corneal pannus. The intraocular lesion treated by couching (which today we call cataract) was actually referred to in Latin as *suffusio*, in the tradition of Celsus, or, beginning possibly as early as the 5th century, as *cataracta*.[16] The drawings might depict a rod scraping a spot off the ocular surface, as opposed to cataract surgery. Moreover, the fact that a picture is dutifully copied does not mean that the action depicted really occurs in the manuscript's era. These eye surgery figures are abstract and stylized.

---

14 No author listed, Sloane 1975, folio 93, at the British Library.

15 No author listed, Harley 1585, folio 9v.

16 Leffler et al. "British Isles" 2021.

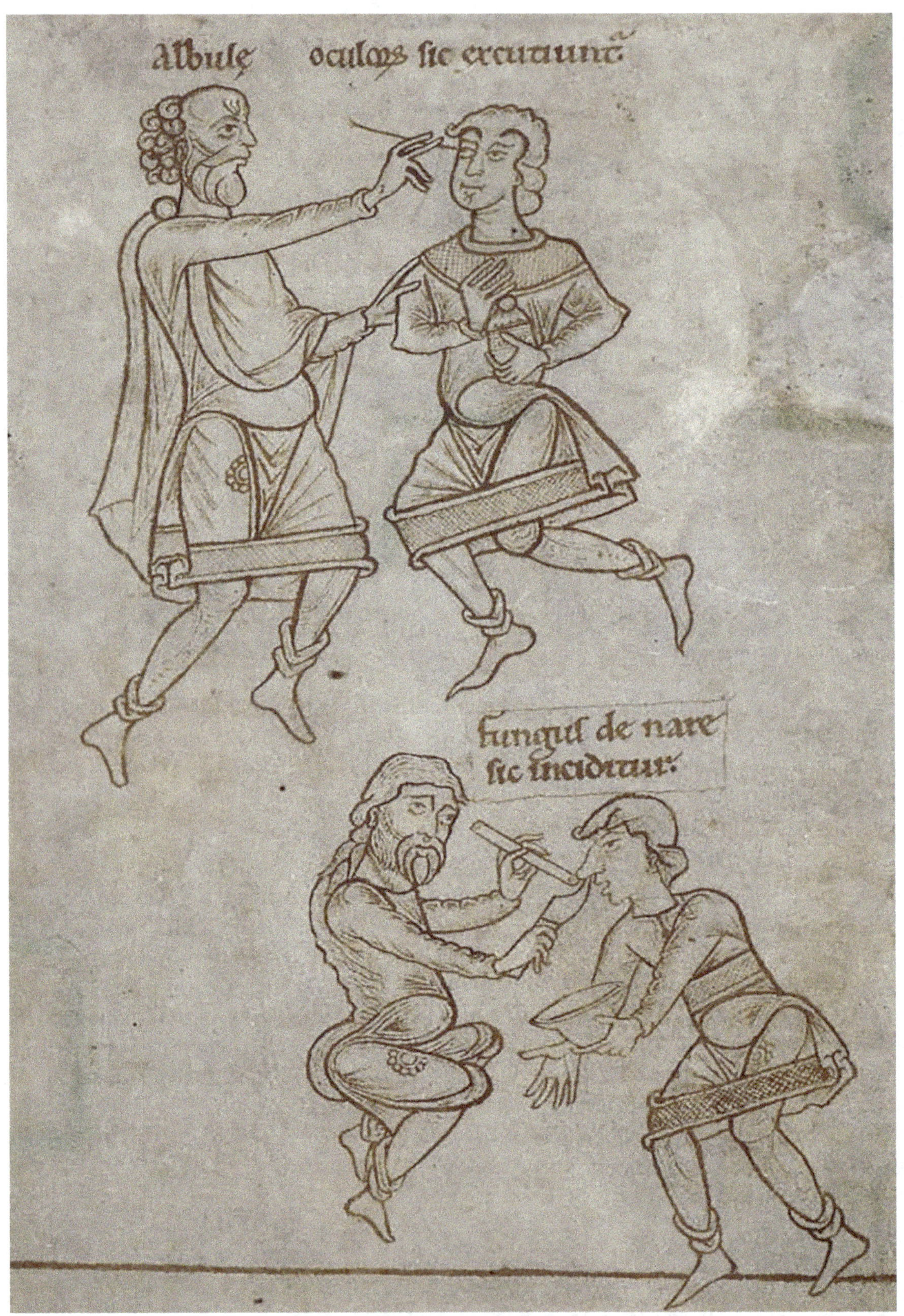

Fig. 3. Harley 1585, a manuscript of the 3rd third quarter of the 12th century, from either the Mosan region of the Netherlands, or England

Knowledge of Couching in Pre-Elizabethan England (1314-1557)

John of Gaddesden (1314)

John of Gaddesden (c. 1280-1349) was an English physician who wrote the medical treatise *Rosa anglica*, which is generally believed to have been composed between 1314 and 1317. As Gaddesden is unaccounted for between 1307 and 1316, Talbot has suggested that this would be a time when Gaddesden could have studied abroad. Indeed, there is some evidence that Gaddesden trained at Montpellier (France). It is interesting that the *Rosa anglica* is thought to have been written toward the end of the time that Gaddesden might have been studying in Montpellier, raising the possibility that it reflects the teachings and experience acquired in that region.

Gaddesden indicated that he had seen cataract couching but did not specify whether his exposure was in England or on the Continent:

> But if the physician or surgeon knows how to cure it [cataract], he will obtain high fees, for it is a common ailment. And I have seen men doing wonders with a needle, so that they were held in high esteem and received more money for one cure of cataract than for ten other diseases.[17]

Gaddesden also described the procedure:

> The patient should sit in front of the physician in a well-lighted place whilst the sun is shining and there is no shadow. His knees should be drawn up to his chest, and bound together, so that he is almost lying down. Then he should look at the end of his nose, opening the eye that is affected: meanwhile the assistant should hold his head, bent back slightly and lift up the eye-lid. Then take the instrument or a steel needle with a round, sharp head, and begin to pierce from the side of lachrymal gland in the conjunctiva pressing it towards the pupil, beginning from the corner of the eye, and let him pierce until he comes to the covering and the pupil between the two tunicles, penetrating to the empty space of the eye which is in front of the pupil. And let the surgeon hold the eye until the perforation is complete, and press the needle down until it is hidden beneath the cornea.[18]

Gaddesden mentioned having the patient turn the operative eye medially, an idea found in Antyllus, and transmitted through the medieval Arabic works. Although Gaddesden appears not to have performed cataract surgery, he did perform other procedures. He removed a stone from under his father's tongue and performed

---

17 Talbot 1967, p. 114.
18 Talbot 1967, p. 114.

bleeding (phlebotomy), setting bones, drawing teeth, cutting corns, and killing lice. Gaddesden died in 1349, probably of the plague.[19]

John of Arderne (1377)

John of Arderne (1307-1392) may have trained and practiced with the military overseas but had returned to England by the time of the Black Death epidemic of 1348. He was best known for performing and reporting surgery for fistula-in-ano. He wrote a treatise on eye diseases, *De Cura Oculorum*, which did not mention cataract surgery.[20] Arderne's ophthalmic work cited Lanfranc of Milan; therefore, Arderne had the opportunity to review what was known about cataract and its surgical treatment. Instead, the only eye conditions specified by Arderne were pannus (*panum*), which he viewed as synonymous with macula (*maculam*), nonspecific terms for white spots on the cornea, ulcer (*ulcera*), and eye inflammation (*lippitudo*).[21] All the eye treatments were essentially medical, though he did recommend phlebotomy from the forehead vein. The detailing of Anglo-Saxon ophthalmic ingredients, which were locally available, and sometimes described in the local vernacular, suggests that the treatise was a practical guide that had been adapted for local use. The only personal experiences were mention of a man whose eye protruded onto his cheek after he was struck with a sword but was successfully treated with a poultice. In addition, Arderne mentioned that a lotion maintained his own eyes at the age of 70, despite extensive studying and writing.[22]

Others were known for treating eye diseases in medieval England. John of Scarborough, active at the end of the 14th century, was known for curing eye diseases, but he is described as a physician, rather than a surgeon. Peter Blank, a surgeon, had legal action taken against him for by a stationer named Simon Lynde in about 1495 for failing to adequately treat the diseased eye of a child.[23]

Treatise of Lanfranc of Milan (1380)

Lanfranc studied under William of Saliceto (in Italy) and brought his methods to France. Lanfranc's surgical treatise of 1296 was translated into Middle English.[24] Lanfranc described cataracts as water falling into the eye:

---

19 Leffler et al. "British Isles" 2021.

20 James 2013, p. 41-46.

21 James 2013, p. 42-45, 247; Schwartz & Leffler 2014.

22 James 2013, p. 45.

23 Leffler et al. "British Isles" 2021.

24 Leffler et al. "British Isles" 2021. Ashmole MS (c. 1380) and the British Museum Additional MS 12,056 (c. 1420). The text from these manuscripts was published for scholars in 1894.

> Cateracta. is water þat falliþ doun bitwixe þe .ij. skynnes of þe iȝe & abidiþ tofore
> þe place þat is clepid pupilla, þat is þe poynt of þe iȝe. & þan it defendiþ þat a man
> mai not se; & it is clepid cataracta.[25]

This 1380 use of the term "cataracta" is the earliest known use of the word in English. Lanfranc's treatise was published in English by surgeon John Hall in 1565. However, Lanfranc's original treatise had details regarding cataract surgery that were not included in the 1565 publication. Lanfranc stated that the patient fasts preoperatively and sits on a stool during the procedure while the surgeon sits a little higher. The nonoperative eye is bound shut, the surgeon chews fennel and blows on the eye, and the couching instrument is made of silver. If the cataract returns, one repeats the depression with the needle. The 1565 edition did not include any of these details. Hall began by noting that one would have to learn the details of cataract surgery from personal observation. Of note, by 1562, Hall knew of and respected the oculist John Luke of London.

Treatise of Benevenutus Grassus (c. 1400)

Another early ophthalmic treatise translated into Middle English was written by Benevenutus Grassus, an eye surgeon plausibly argued to be from a Jewish family, and who might have spent time in Salerno, Jerusalem, and Montpellier. He is thought to date from the first half of the 13th century. Grassus' detailed understanding of couching has led historians to believe that he actually performed the procedure. His Latin treatise was one of the first medical texts to be printed in 1474. Several versions of Grassus' work in Middle or early modern English are of interest. The earliest manuscript dates from the first half of the 15th century, but only has portions of the treatise. The surviving portions use the term "cataractes" when referencing Grassus' discussion of the disorder: "...we did nedill it after þe maner of agulying as it is taught aboue in doctrine of cataractes and so he was clenelich y heled and clerely he toke and recouered his siȝt..."[26] Corresponding text in the other Middle English manuscripts indicates that this patient was a child of Messana (Messina, Sicily) who developed a cataract after a ruptured globe.[27] Middle English versions of Grassus' treatise are found in manuscripts from the mid-15th century onward.[28] In 1583, an English version of Grassus treatise was incorporated in Philip Barrough's *Method of Physick* and was frequently republished in various medical works for the next 70 years.[29] In 1590, surgeon Joseph Fenton produced his own version of Grassus' treatise. Fenton added marginal notes, disparaging Barrough's translation.[30]

---

25 Leffler et al. "British Isles" 2021.

26 Grassus 2011, p. 405.

27 Grassus 2011, p. 408-409.

28 Grassus 2011, pp. 42, 168.

29 Leffler et al. "Elizabethan" 2014.

30 Grassus 2011, p. 168. Fenton's manuscript is British Library Sloane MS 661. Grassus' method is in an earlier chapter in this volume.

The Middle English manuscripts do not use the term "couching" to describe the procedure, but Fenton's 1590 version does use the term. In addition, a late 1400s copyist of the treatise introduced an error, because he did not realize that cataract surgeons were supposed to be ambidextrous. This error was corrected by surgeon Joseph Fenton when he copied the manuscript in 1590.[31] These English manuscripts of Grassus' treatise are consistent with the actual practice of cataract surgery being unfamiliar in England before the 15th century but established by the Elizabethan period.

Treatise of Guy de Chauliac (1425)

Guy de Chauliac (c. 1300-1368) was one of the preeminent surgical authors of the 14th century. He trained in 1325 at Montpellier and also at Bologna and Paris. In 1363, while at Avignon, he wrote a surgical treatise in Latin, his *Chirugia Magna*, also called the *Inventarium*. One Middle English translation, known as the *Inventorye*, is found in a manuscript, which dates from about 1425. An independent Middle English translation, known as the Cyrugie, used the term "catharacta" or "catheractes" to describe the fully developed form of cataract.[32] In Chauliac's couching description, the surgeon blows on the eye, and the patient turns the eye toward the nose. Chauliac noted that others preferred a gold or silver needle, but he preferred iron, as it was less likely to break. Chauliac's 1363 use of the term "oculistas" in Latin was translated into Middle English in about 1425 as "oculisterz."[33]

Balthasar Guercy (1519)

Balthasar Guercy (d. 1557), of Italy, was trained in medicine on the continent and arrived in England in about 1515. Two separate lines of evidence might link Guercy with cataract surgery: (1) the use of the term "couching" by his rival Thomas Roos and (2) Guercy's treatment of the eye of archbishop and royal advisor Cardinal Thomas Wolsey.

Guercy's opponent, surgeon Thomas Roos, felt threatened by the understanding of anatomy and physiology that Guercy had acquired overseas. Guercy complained to Katherine and then to King Henry VIII that Roos was harassing him. On November 7, 1519, Guercy was granted an injunction against Roos, who was fined 100 pounds and ordered "not to molest Balthazar…or pursue information late put into the King's Exchequer, till he proves that surgery is a handicraft." In his response, Roos defined surgery as including "..cuttyng of the sculle in due proporcyon to the pellicules of the brayne with instruments of iron, cowchyng of catharacts, takying owt bonys, sowying of the flesshe, launching of bocchis, cutting of apostumes…letting of blo[o]

---

31 Leffler et al. "British Isles" 2021.
32 Leffler et al. "British Isles" 2021.
33 Leffler et al. "British Isles" 2021.

d, drawying of te[e]the…which restyth onely in manuall operation…"[34] Roos' 1519 use of the term "cowchying" to describe cataract surgery is the earliest surviving instance (to our knowledge).

Cardinal Thomas Wolsey (1473-1530) received treatment for an eye disorder, at least a portion of which was provided by Guercy. John Skelton's 1522 poem *Why Come ye nat to Courte* suggested that Guercy's treatment of Cardinal Wolsey's eye would render him blind.

> With a flap afore his eye / Men wene that he is pocky / Or els[e] his surgions they lye / For as far as the[y] can spy / By the craft of surgery / It is manus domini… / That all his trust hangis / In Balthasor [Guercy] / whiche he[a]led / Domi[n]gos nose / that was wheled… / Balthasor [Guercy] y he[a]lyd domi[n]gos nose / From the puskyde pocky pose / Now with his gumys of araby / Hath [pro]mised to he[a]le our cardinals [Wolsey's] eye / Yet sum surgio[n]s put a dou[b]t / Lest he wyll put it cle[a]ne out.[35]

Skelton's suggestion that Wolsey's eye was "pocky" would typically suggest syphilis but might occasionally refer to smallpox. The suggestion that a surgeon would put an eye out was exactly the criticism rendered toward later cataract surgeons not accepted by the mainstream, such as Valentine Russwurin (discussed later). Skelton's summary of Wolsey's condition in Latin translates as:

> Oppressed with the Neapolitan disease [syphilis], laid low under plaster poultices, pierced by the surgeon's iron instrument [*Pharmacapoli ferro foratum*], relieved by nothing, nor made better by any medicine…[36]

Piercing would describe cataract surgery better than a procedure to scrape a corneal spot off the eye. The flap has been thought by some to indicate disfigurement from the disease, such as ptosis, but this line by Skelton is actually listed in the Oxford English Dictionary to define flap as "anything that hangs broad and loose, fastened only by one side."[37] This definition would be consistent with an eye patch. A Spanish message from 1522 confirmed some sort of systemic problem affecting the eye of Wolsey, who was "so very ill that he is in danger of losing an eye, and the rest of his body seems almost equally affected."[38]

Treatise of Giovanni da Vigo (1543)

Giovanni da Vigo (c. 1450-1525) practiced in Genoa, Savona, and Rome. His major surgical work was published in 1514. Its English translation was published by

---

34 Leffler et al. "British Isles" 2021.

35 Leffler et al. "British Isles" 2021.

36 Leffler et al. "British Isles" 2021.

37 Leffler et al. "British Isles" 2021.

38 Leffler et al. "British Isles" 2021.

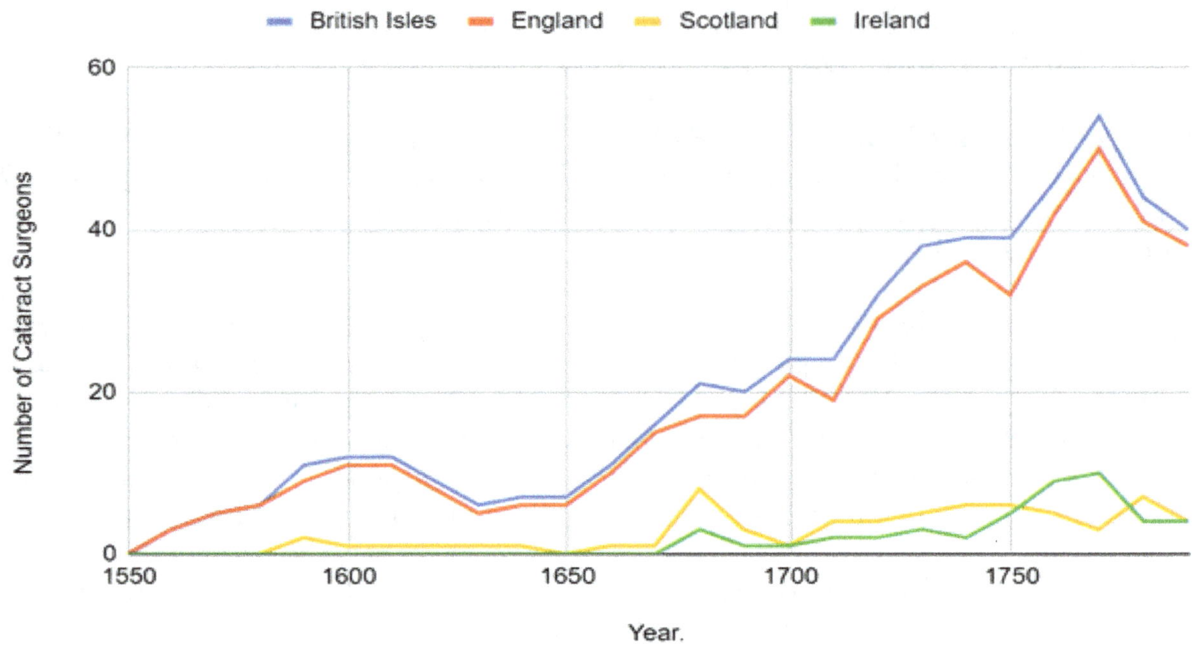

Fig. 4. Number of probable cataract surgeons in the British Isles, for each decade (1550-1800).

Bartholomew Traheron (c. 1510-1558) in 1543. Vigo wrote that the typical surgeon would not perform cataract surgery—it was left to "ye to[o]th drawers" (dentists).[39]

Elizabethan Cataract Surgeons (1558-1603)

John Luke of London (1561)

In the Elizabethan era, we find stronger evidence of cataract surgeons in the British Isles, beginning with England (Fig. 4). John Luke of London was licensed by the Royal College of Physicians to treat eye diseases in 1561. The College stipulated that he was restricted to using external medicines. No internal medicines or enemas could be used. No mention of surgery was made, but perhaps the physicians did not care to regulate procedures that did not encroach upon their clinical territory.[40]

Luke seems to have made quite a splash in London at this time and was respected by eminent surgeons and physicians. The 1562 lectures of physician William Bullein noted: "Of Foenigreke is an excellent Fomentum made for the iyen [eyes], that be

---

39 Leffler et al. "British Isles" 2021.

40 Leffler et al. "British Isles" 2021.

sore or dim: which I have seen mayster Luke make, which is an excellent man, in the cure or Regiment for the eyes." A footnote specifies "Maister Luke of London."[41]

Surgeon John Hall recounted another story from 1562 in which a shoemaker from Kent named William said that he could cure "sore eyes": "And that whereas maister Luke of London, hath a great name of curing eyes: he could do that which maister Luke could not do, nor turn his hand to." The shoemaker bragged that he could do some type of eye surgery which Luke could not. Hall called Luke "that reverent man of known learning and experience" and demonstrated that the shoemaker knew no eye anatomy.[42]

Banister grants Luke priority among English "Oculistes": "The first and cheifest was Luke of Erithe [in London] a man that lived in great fame and credit had the greatest practice and sums of money for he hath had from XX to LX L for Cataracke couchinge."[43] If this attribution of priority is correct, then Luke probably was couching in the early 1560s. It is thought that Luke might be the author of several anti-papist satirical tracts published about 1548 under the name Luke Shepherd.[44] Shepherd was born in Colchester and was imprisoned at least briefly for his writings. Luke, the oculist of London, made money from a "diet drink," required patients to lie on their backs for 9 days postoperatively, and occasionally practiced in an itinerant manner.[45] It is not clear that Luke took any apprentices, as Banister remembered "all his knowledge was buried with him." Luke "died at London at Mr Best's house in ye stocks."[46]

Thomas Surflet (1560s)

Thomas Surflet (1531-1611) was probably one of the earliest couchers after Luke. In his published treatise, Banister listed "Master Surflet of Lynne" as among his "most skillful" advisors who were "all excelling in the operations."[47] But in his un-published manuscript, Banister told a different story about "…Mr. Surphlete, a man of excellent Diet and crusty fashion of body. He lived till he was four score years of age, lived most in Norfolke, & died at Linn, and in good estate…I cannot commend this Mr. Surphlete for any extraordinary skill, though of long experience."[48] Skillful or not, it seems Surflet was an important early ophthalmic teacher.

In 1559, one Thomas Surflet was granted a license to practice surgery by Cambridge University on the basis of many years of the study and practice of surgery.

---

41 Leffler et al. "British Isles" 2021.

42 Leffler et al. "British Isles" 2021.

43 James 2013, pp. 51-55.

44 Leffler et al. "British Isles" 2021.

45 James 2013, p. 53.

46 James 2013, p. 54.

47 Banister 1971, np.

48 James 2013.

Between 1564 and 1577, Thomas Surflet owned a property in Peterborough. Thus, Surflet might have taught Banister's advisor "Master Barnabie of Peter-Borough." If so, then Surflet might have been performing couching by the early 1560s. William Barnaby was married at St. John's Church in Peterborough in 1568. When Barnaby was buried there in 1600, he was remembered as "a good Townsman."[49]

Surflet became a freeman in Lynn in 1579 and was required to treat the poor for free at the request of the mayor. Banister recorded that at Lynn, Surflet "lay 2 or 3 years at a barber's house at Linn to whom he taught some skill, who now professeth it with weak Understanding and given to drink."[50] We argue that this barber was probably author Richard Seabrooke (see later).

In 1589, Robert Greve (or Greene) was listed as an apprentice to Surflet in Lynn. Greene was excommunicated in 1597 for practicing surgery without a license.

A younger surgeon named Richard Surflet (c. 1560-1604) knew how to couch cataracts and, because of the shared surname, is assumed to have learned from the elder Surflet. In 1599, Richard Surflet translated into English: *A discourse of the preservation of the sight: of melancholike diseases: of rheumes, and of old age*, originally written by André Du Laurens. In the preface, Surflet wrote: "Which Surphlet famous for his art-taught cunning hand, In clearing the Eyes of spots, and noisome Catarrhacts..." and also "Surphlet...famous for thy art, In curing of blind catarrhacted eyes." In 1604, Richard Surflet sailed for the East Indies as a ship's physician and preacher, but he died on the return voyage.[51]

Valentine Russwurin (1573)

Although cataract surgery by Englishmen in the 1560s is suggested by reports from several decades later, by the 1570s, we begin to see contemporaneously documented records of immigrants performing the surgery. Queen Elizabeth reigned from 1558 until her death in 1603. We know that she was aware of the German surgeon Valentine Russwurin, of Schmalkalden. Russwurin had previously practiced at Königsberg, Hamburg, and Groningen. The earliest reference to Russwurin in London is thought to be the report of an "Allmaigne [German] surgeon" in the letter from August 29, 1573, of William Herle to William Cecil.[52] Herle's job was to gather intelligence for Cecil, the chief advisor to the queen. Herle did not use the language that became typical of the Elizabethan era because that language had not yet evolved. Herle did not describe Russwurin as an oculist. Rather, Herle called Russwurin "the new surgion opthalmist."[53] Likewise, Herle never used the term "cataract" to describe the visual disorder of the patients, or the term "couching" to

---

49 Leffler et al. "British Isles" 2021.

50 James 2013, p. 54.

51 Leffler et al. "British Isles" 2021.

52 Leffler et al. "British Isles" 2021.

53 Leffler et al. "British Isles" 2021.

describe the procedure. Russwurin's techniques were new enough that they merited report to the Queen's deputy.

Russwurin performed at least some treatments at the patients' house, but he advertised his services from a market stall he set up outside London's Royal Exchange.[54] Russwurin "had restored one Jone Wynter a widow to her sight, who hath been blind these 8 years, & is of the age of 66 years…"[55] Herle reported that in Russwurin's hands, "…after some handling of her eye, what with instrument & otherwise, & then applying some juices & powder to the same, had made her to see in an instant well nye & to discern his face & chain of gold perfectly, with another color that was presented. But when the sight is thus restored, he accustoms to diet his patients & to keep them with plasters out of the air to confirm the tenderness of their sight for a month or 6 weeks after this cure: having now in cure at his own house within Bisshops gate street, on Ales Burton…who was blind, of the one eye 2 yeres, & of the other eye 3 weekes, & hath made her to see with that speed & facility which he did the other…."[56]

Russwurin described himself as an "Opthalmiste" and noted that "there were some causes & effect of blindness…that were utterly incurable."[57] Russwurin set up a stall at the Royal Exchange in London where he advertised his services. He displayed bladder stones, which he had removed, and provided testimonials from patients whom he had surgically treated for cataracts. He advocated the medical ideas of Paracelsus. In a letter to William Cecil, Russwurin discussed Cecil's mother's cataracts, especially the hard "tartar" in cataracts, and indicated that he could treat Cecil's mother.[58] The letter is undated but must have been written before 1587, when Cecil's mother died. In fact, the letter was probably written before May 1574, when Russwurin was run out of town. Russwurin's letter of 1573 or 1574 about Cecil's mother is the earliest known use of the term cataract with reference to a specific English patient, even if locals like Herle did not adopt the term at that time. It is not known if Russwurin ultimately treated Cecil's mother, but she was blind by December 1574. Russwurin's time in London peaked when he was made a "denizen" by Elizabeth in early 1574. However, Russwurin's status rapidly spiraled downward. From the beginning, according to Herle, "…the Physicians & Surgeons do envy this [Russwurin's practice], & have used many ways & speeches to deface him."[59] William Clowes, a member of the St. Bartholomew's hospital staff, derided "Valentine Rarsworme, of Smalcalde, a stranger born" for claiming the titles "of Medicus Spagiricus, chirurgus, Lithotomus, and Opthalmiste."[60] In more than one patient, Russwurin tried to surgically extract bladder stones, but when no stone

---

54 Leffler et al. "British Isles" 2021.

55 Leffler et al. "British Isles" 2021.

56 Leffler et al. "British Isles" 2021.

57 Leffler et al. "British Isles" 2021.

58 Leffler et al. "British Isles" 2021.

59 Leffler et al. "British Isles" 2021.

60 Leffler et al. "British Isles" 2021.

was to be found, he surreptitiously retrieved a stone already in his possession and pretended it had come from the patient. According to Clowes, many of Russwurin's lithotomy patients died. Russwurin also unsuccessfully treated an ophthalmic ailment in Andrew Castleton (d. 1617), a deacon at Cambridge, who ultimately was remembered as being blind.[61] The treatments of Wynter, Burton, and Castleton appear consistent with cataract couching. If so, they would be the earliest identified patients to undergo couching in England. After all of these clinical misadventures, a trial at Guild Hall was conducted in May 1574. Seeing that a pillory was being erected for him, Russwurin "doubting the worst, and to prevent the same, upon a sudden he hid his head…"[62] Presumably, Russwurin absconded.

Richard Seabrooke (1579)

Richard Seabrooke (1548-1624) of King's Lynn wrote the earliest ophthalmic treatise by an English oculist. As noted earlier, Seabrooke is likely the Lynn barber mentioned by Banister and was taught by Thomas Surflet about 1579. Seabrooke's age of about 30 years upon Surflet's arrival in the town would be consistent with his writing (at the age of 72): "being from my youth by profession an Occulist…," Seabrooke shared patients with "M. Surfleet, a very skillful Occulist."[63]

In a 14-month-old infant who had lost vision, Surflet thought treatment was futile, but Seabrooke saw no harm in having the nursing mother regularly drink ale infused with eyebright (euphrasia), betony, and fennel. Seabrooke gathered herbs himself in May or June and dried them for use throughout the year.

Just as Seabrooke was willing to disagree with Surflet about this case, he was also willing to disagree with the medical profession more generally about the effect of therapeutic bleeding. The student of history often wonders why clinicians could not discern that bleeding made patients worse. In fact, Seabrooke did figure that out. He saw no benefit and in fact described patients who went blind after bleeding. Seabrooke practiced not far from Richard Banister, and the patients' hometowns were close to those of both oculists. For instance, there was "Goodman Fletcher, dwelling in a little Town near Bourne in Lincolne Shiere, having some small impediment in his eyes, and coming to an ignorant Practitioner, had a vein opened in his temples, and another by his nose, but the blood was no sooner received, when as the sight was utterly lost forever."[64] It is likely that some of these patients were treated by Banister. As noted earlier, Banister returned the favor by describing Seabrooke as an alcoholic with a weak understanding.

As with Russwurin, Seabrooke determined the curability of a "Catharack" by its color. The curable cataracts were hazel, "the color of the sky," and "grayish." The

---

61 Leffler et al. "British Isles" 2021.
62 Leffler et al. "British Isles" 2021.
63 Leffler et al. "British Isles" 2021.
64 Leffler et al. "British Isles" 2021.

incurable cataracts were black, white, and "yellowish green." If the patient could not see sunlight or candlelight, there was no hope. Seabrooke did not divulge the specifics of how these were "cured by the Catharack needle" because he believed only trained experts should attempt the surgery. The patient must lie down for 8 or 9 days postoperative to prevent the cataract from rising.

To Seabrooke, "the Pin and the Web" represented small white corneal opacities, which were treated with eye drops made from honey, daisies, and woman's milk. Scarring from "small Pocks" (smallpox) was treated by blowing a powder made from "white Sugar-candy." For a "filme" upon the eye, one applied eye drops made from "the marrow of a Goose wing" mixed with powdered ginger. If an injury thrust the eye onto the cheek, he pushed the eye back for several hours and then applied a dressing of breadcrumbs mixed with milk. The doctor could also blow into the eye, provided he did not eat garlic or use tobacco ahead of time.

For difficulty reading at near in the older adult, he recommended the powder taken in ale. Young students with difficulty reading fine print could use the powder taken orally in ale, or a hat to protect them from the light. He did not mention spectacles or magnifying glasses.

Overall, Seabrooke's treatments were above average for the period. He had many years of experience as an oculist and performed couching. His greatest accomplishment was figuring out that therapeutic bleeding is harmful. He did not totally get away from harsh treatments, such as blistering, purging, and enemas, but he did not emphasize these. His practice included both the gentle ale-based medicines of royal physician Walter Bailey and, when indicated, the newer technique of couching.[65]

Early Cataract Patients (1581)

For some early cataract patients, the surgeon who performed or considered cataract surgery is unknown. Edmund Grindal (c. 1519–1583), the archbishop of Canterbury, had declining vision by 1581, and Queen Elizabeth suggested that he resign. Grindal was close with the queen's advisor, William Cecil, to whom the exiled Russwurin's ophthalmic treatments were reported. Indeed, until the end of 1582, Grindal had some hope of recovering his vision: "…he had before entertained some hope of recovering his sight, as some others in like case had done…"[66] By the end of 1582, however, he accepted the permanence of his blindness. On his stone effigy at Croydon Minster, "his eyes have a kind of white in the pupil to denote his blindness."[67]

---

65 Leffler et al. "Elizabethan" 2014.

66 Leffler et al. "British Isles" 2021.

67 Leffler et al. "British Isles" 2021. Unfortunately, the effigy was destroyed when the church burned in 1867.

Bernardino de Mendoza (c. 1540–1604) arrived in England as the Spanish ambassador in 1578. In 1579, at age 39, he wrote that he had "precoz ceguera" (precocious blindness).[68] In 1583, his poor vision resulted in an accident. In 1584, he was expelled from England, and his king stationed him in Paris. Therefore, he endured at least 5 years of visual difficulties in England, apparently without undergoing any eye surgeries. In 1585, he noted that he had fatigue of the eyes due to "el humor," which had settled in them, causing "dolor" (pain) and "caliente" (heat). In 1586, he had surgery performed with "la aguja" (the needle) for "una catarata" of the left eye while under the care of "los médicos y oculistas" of Paris.[69] Nonetheless, by 1589, he was almost completely blind.

Richard Carew of Cornwall (1555-1620), a translator and antiquary, had bilateral cataract surgery, apparently in about 1615, by an unknown oculist. Carew's use of spectacles after cataract surgery is the first that we know of in England. The fact that the cataract surgery in the second eye at first seemed to fail, but then worked later, could be attributed either to the slow absorption of residual lens cortex or from the lens initially blocking the visual axis, but later dislocating (among other causes).[70]

Physician and astrologer Richard Napier (1559-1634) recorded the cataract couchings of several patients whose surgeon is unknown and, by 1600, used the term "cataract" to describe their condition.[71] Other cataract patients are known, independent of advertisements from the surgeon. Bartholomew Vanderlashe was given permission to perform eye surgery on one Melser Gisberd in 1612.[72] Peter Heylyn (1599-1662), the royal chaplain, had cataracts from 1654 onward, severe enough to require other men to guide him, but the cataracts were considered too immature to couch.[73] George Williamson performed an unsuccessful couching in 1663.[74] Steward Walter Powell (1603-1654), of Wales, was couched in 1653-1654 successively by Mr. Middleton, Anthony Atwood, and Mr. Fayrfax. William Green, of Newcastle, was the "Dr. Green" who unsuccessfully couched the cataract of benefactor Robert

---

68 Leffler et al. "British Isles" 2021.

69 Leffler et al. "British Isles" 2021.

70 Leffler et al. "British Isles" 2021. Also see Dr. Letocha's account of the Carew case elsewhere in this volume.

71 In 1600, Napier referred to William Burnet of Great Horwood having a "cataract of w[hi]ch he was twice cut." On July 7, 1622, Napier asked whether in Goodman Robert Richardson of Newport, Wales, "the Dutchma[n] will recoav[e]r his...eye sight." In that era, "Dutchman" referred to someone from Germany or Holland. Bartholomew Vanderlashe of Germany was indeed couching cataracts in that era. By July 22, 1622, the surgery had been performed: "Richardson...had his eyes opened." Nonetheless, in 1629, Richardson was described as "blynd 7 y[ears] extremely tormented in his left ey[e] w[hi]ch was good for a long tyme & now is tormented" Napier recorded on June 3, 1625, that Nicholas Ridley of Weston, age 74 years, was "cut of on Cataract & doth see by a skilfull oculist" (Leffler et al. "British Isles" 2021).

72 Leffler et al. "British Isles" 2021.

73 Leffler et al. "British Isles" 2021.

74 Leffler & Schwartz "Woolhouse" 2017.

Thomlinson (1668–1748) on July 17, 1736. Minister David Maitland of Aberdeen had been blind for several years, beginning in about 1734 when he was "couched of a cataract by the celebrated Mr. George Lauder, Surgeon [of Edinburg], by which his sight was restored."[75] In 1588, physician and astrologer Simon Forman witnessed a cataract surgery performed by Marian Lerret of France and used the term "cataract" to describe the condition.[76]

Joseph Fenton (1590).

Joseph Fenton (c. 1565/1570-1634) was an Elizabethan surgeon who, in copying and correcting the treatise of Benevenutus Grassus in 1590, introduced the term "couching" to the treatise and demonstrated a keen interest in cataract surgery, as discussed earlier. In July 1607, Fenton was appointed one of the examiners of surgeons for the Barber Company of London. He, therefore, would have examined Mathias Jenkinson (d. 1625) in July 1608, who was "lycenced to cut for the hernia or Rupture to couch the Cat[a]rac[t] to cut for the wry neck & the hare lip" but was required to have a representative of the Company present at "every such Cure." However, in June 1609, Jenkinson was "discharged from his practice in Surgery" for violating the licensure terms "and for his evil & unskillful[l] practice."[77]

Henry Blackborne (1594)

One dynamic ophthalmic teacher of the period was Henry Blackborne (d. 1611), probably born about 1573 in Halifax, Yorkshire. His family might have moved to Kent. Banister painted a mixed picture of "Henry Blackburne who travelled continuously from one market town to another, who could couche ye Cataracke well, cure it, Lay a scar [cleft] Lipe, set a cro[o]ckt necke straight & help deafnesse."[78] On the other hand, Blackborne deceived patients by charging handsomely to treat incurable conditions. Likewise, Blackborne himself was "often deceived of great sums of money but never robbed."[79] Because he was "lusty amorously given to several women," he frequently had to flee and change his name and "was often imprisoned for women."[80] After couching a cataract, Blackborne placed a linen cloth dipped in beaten egg white over the eye, with instructions to change the dressing twice daily

---

75 Leffler et al. "British Isles" 2021.

76 Leffler et al. "British Isles" 2021. According to texts from Italy, Queen Elizabeth summoned the surgeon Cesare Scacchi of Preci to her court just before 1590. Some have suggested this was to perform a cataract surgery on the queen. However, we have reviewed the question in detail and agree with those who have suggested that Scacchi was more likely summoned to deal with the urinary difficulties of the queen's secretary Francis Walsingham (Leffler et al. "British Isles" 2021).

77 Leffler et al. "British Isles" 2021.

78 James 2013, p. 54.

79 James 2013, p. 55.

80 James 2013, p. 54.

for 9 days. He only returned for a postoperative visit if he heard that the patient had done well.[81]

Blackborne taught an apothecary named Page, who never acquired much skill. The first surgeon Blackborne instructed in cataract couching was named Hanle. Hanle also practiced in an itinerant manner and conflicted with his teacher over who had the bigger practice. Hanle also operated on cataracts before they were ready and was once beaten by an unsatisfied patient. If patients could not see after 9 days, they would demand their money back, so Hanle moved along before the bandages came off the eye. Hanle had no academic understanding of disease, according to Banister, but "For couching of Cataracke he would do it exellent well."[82] Banister met Hanle when Hanle visited Sleaford and set up "his show" in the market, and only later did Banister meet Blackborne at York. Banister probably began practicing at Sleaford in the early 1600s.

Banister informs us that "Blackburne instructed one Nelson that married his sister. He could couche the Cataracke well but was given to drunkeness & so died beggarly."[83] Blackborne's sister married John Nelson of York, "Chirurgeon" in Bishopsbourne, Kent, in 1596. Blackborne had married into the Nelson family of York in 1594. Nelson's listing as a surgeon suggests that Blackborne had already begun teaching by 1596.[84]

One "Blackborne" of Canterbury was granted a license to practice surgery on June 4, 1594. On August 17, 1605, Henry Blackborne was licensed to cure eye diseases in Canterbury. On September 7, 1610, the mayor of Rye in Sussex provided a certificate for Henry Blackborne, "chirurgion and occulist" for curing the blind of Rye 1 year before: "by…his art and skill, did recover diverse persons…that were blinde, unto their sight again."[85] Blackborne treated a 74-year-old widow "darke and blinde" for 2 years and 65- and 75-year-old wives of two fishermen, one of whom had been "blinde" for 10 years.[86] The lengthy duration speaks to the lack of availability of couching. All three patients "can see, and go about the town without any guide."[87] Blackborne described himself as an "Oculist" of Edgware, Middlesex, in his will, probated in 1611. Banister remembered that he "died in Kent".[88]

---

81 James 2013, p. 54.

82 James 2013, p. 56.

83 James 2013, p. 55.

84 Leffler et al. "British Isles" 2021.

85 Leffler et al. "British Isles" 2021.

86 Leffler et al. "British Isles" 2021.

87 Leffler et al. "British Isles" 2021.

88 Leffler et al. "British Isles" 2021.

James Van Otten (c. 1601)

James Van Otten (1568-1622), of Ypres (Belgium), was born in 1568 and received a medical degree from Leiden University in 1593. He was present in England by 1601 and began training apprentices. Some time about 1601, he trained Richard Banister.[89]

Nicholas Bowden (1576-1649), another Van Otten apprentice, was born in Loughborough, Leicestershire. In 1601, Van Otten and Bowden were jointly permitted by the Company of Barber Surgeons to practice in London "only for the couchinge of the catarack, cutting for the rupture [hernia], stone, and wenne [boil]."[90] Moreover, "Bowden shall be assistant unto the said James Vanotten."[91] In return, the surgeons were required to pay a fee to the Company, which would be used for the poor. They could hang an advertising banner at their lodging, but nowhere else.

In 1602, Bowden was licensed by the University of Cambridge to practice surgery. By about 1605, Bowden advertised as a "Chirurgion, cutter of the stone, and also Occulest, curer of the Ruptures [hernias] without cutting..."[92] Bowden also treated "all hare or cleft lips." With respect to vision, he promised: "All Rumes, pearles, blemishes, or Catteracts curable, although they have been long blind, they shall in short time receive sight."[93] In 1614, "Nicholas Bowden" was "certified fit by the professor" and licensed to practice surgery by Oxford University.[94] In July 1648, Bowden gave a manuscript on alchemy to antiquarian Elias Ashmole. Bowden, described as "Master of Chirurgiens," was buried in Reading on December 24, 1649.[95]

In November 1607, Van Otten recommended the otherwise unknown Mr. Charles to couch a cataract. By 1619, Van Otten had a new favorite oculist, when Napier recorded: "Atwood of Worcester a gentlema[n] of 500 ll [libra] the ye[a]re & the best Co [sic] Oculist in England comēnded by Mr Van Otten."[96] It is interesting that Van Otten preferred Atwood to Van Otten's former students Banister and Bowden. Whether Atwood was trained by Van Otten is not known. Atwood was ultimately the patriarch of a family with five generations of oculists between 1619 and 1751, including luminaries such as John Stepkins and John Thomas Woolhouse.[97]

In May 1620, when the teacher Van Otten was licensed to practice surgery by the University of Oxford, he was hailed as "a very learned expert chirurgian well

---

89 Leffler et al. "British Isles" 2021.

90 Leffler et al. "British Isles" 2021.

91 Leffler et al. "British Isles" 2021.

92 Leffler et al. "British Isles" 2021.

93 Leffler et al. "British Isles" 2021.

94 Leffler et al. "British Isles" 2021.

95 Leffler et al. "British Isles" 2021.

96 Leffler et al. "British Isles" 2021.

97 Leffler & Schwartz "Woolhouse" 2017.

practiced in the faculty these thirty years in his own country, this, and other king-doms."[98] He was matriculated as a privileged person at Oxford on April 6, 1621.

In 1619, Van Otten took an apprentice named Percivall Willughby, in return for receiving £100 for 7 years. However, Van Otten died in 1622. Under the heading: "On the death of Mr. James Van Otten an expert Chirurgion, who dyed att Oxford: March: 1. 1622," poet William Strode remembered: "Death now growes politique:/ While Otton liv'd herselfe was weake and sicke/ For want of food, therefore at him she aimde...Behold Death's triumph and our fatall losse."[99]

Richard Banister (c. 1602)

Richard Banister (c. 1570-1626) has been called the father of British ophthalmology, primarily because his 1622 ophthalmic treatise contained some novel and important observations, and was influential enough to be republished almost a century later.[100]

He spent 5 or 6 years studying under his uncle, surgeon and anatomist John Ban-ister (1533-1610).[101] It seems the elder Banister always had some interest in the eyes. In 1570, John Banister had confirmed the finding of Italian anatomist Realdo Colombo that the "watrish" (aqueous) humor would reform after its loss through a wound to the eye. In 1578, John Banister also reported the correct teaching of Realdo Colombo that the lens is anteriorly positioned, in contrast with the fallacy dating from the medieval Arabic period that the lens is positioned in the exact center of the eye. In 1578, John Banister noted the changing ophthalmic terminology among younger practitioners: In the anterior chamber, "...suffusions are made, which the younger sort have called Cataractes."[102] John Banister knew of Grassus' treatise through its republication by Philip Barrough and also gave Guillemeau's 1585 ophthalmic treatise to Anthony Hunton, whose English translation was published in 1587 (Fig. 5).[103]

Given this ophthalmic interest, some have looked to John Banister as the source of Richard Banister's ophthalmic knowledge. However, Banister was clear in his book's dedication that what he learned from his uncle was general surgery.[104] After the time with his uncle, Richard Banister spent a year or 2 in the chamber of "Lorde Willaby." Banister recounted, "then I spent a little tyme (with) one James of Utricke in ye Lowe C[o]untryes."[105] Given that James Van Otten of Utrecht was in England training apprentices who subsequently couched cataracts, Van Otten would seem

---

98 Leffler et al. "British Isles" 2021.

99 Leffler et al. "British Isles" 2021.

100 Banister 1971.

101 James 2013, p. 57.

102 Leffler et al. "British Isles" 2021.

103 Leffler et al. "Elizabethan" 2014.

104 Leffler et al. "British Isles" 2021.

105 James 2013, p. 57.

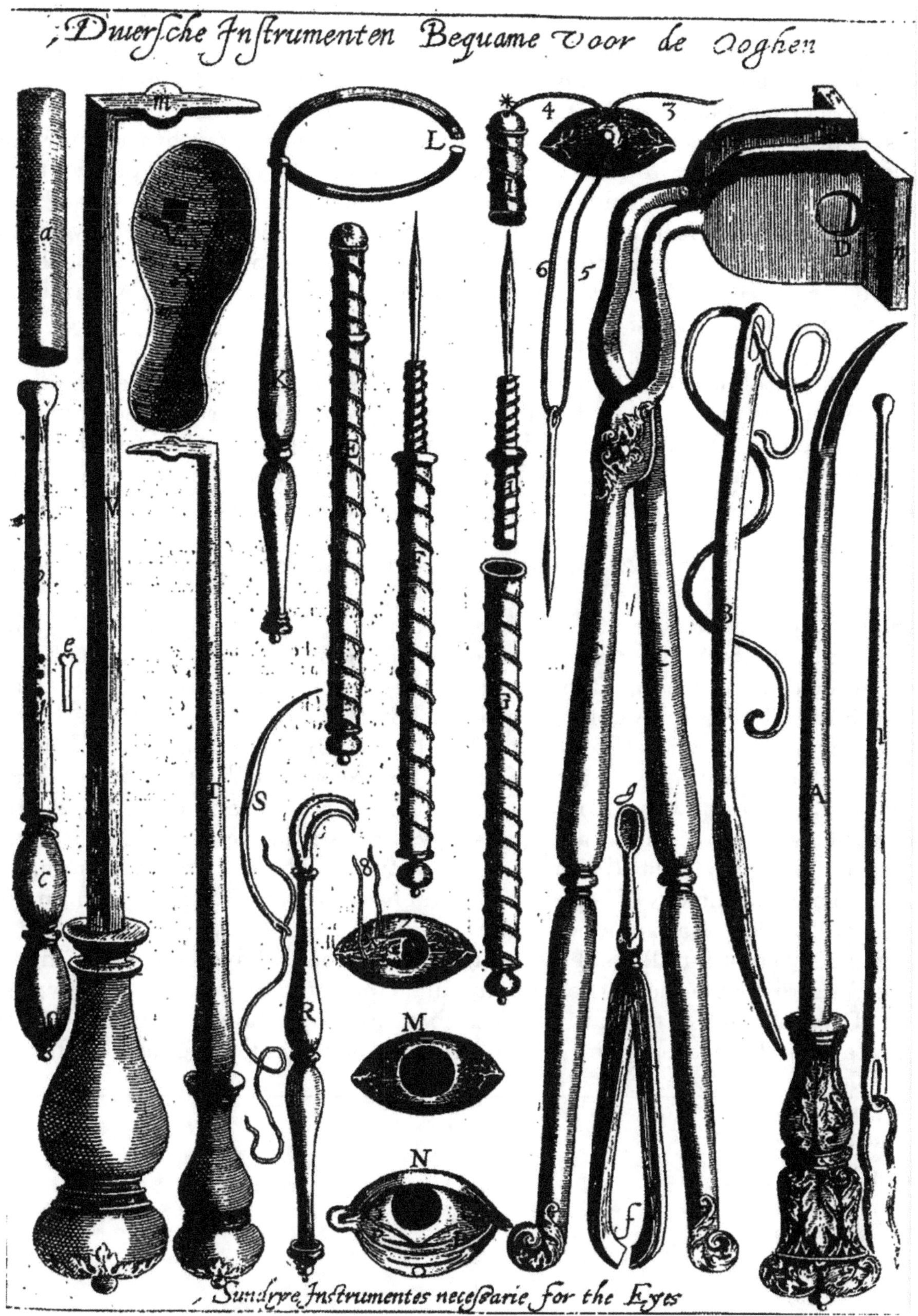

Fig. 5. Eye instruments, including "the Needle to remove the Cataractes" from the 1598 translation of Jacque Guillemeau's *The Frenche chirurgerye.*

to be Banister's mentor. Banister then spent 14 years practicing at Sleaford. Given that he was licensed to practice surgery in Sleaford in 1602, his training with Van Otten would probably been around 1601.[106] Richard Banister decided to specialize in order to perfect his practice. He was interested in eyesight after "finding some defects in mine owne eyes."[107] He also performed "helpe of Hearing by the instrument, the cure of the Hare-lip, and the wry Necke. When in the threshold of my practice, I could couch the Cataract, and so began to gaine some name of an Oculist."[108] Perhaps, Banister had a falling out with Van Otten, because Banister only spent "a little tyme" with Van Otten and also failed to mention Van Otten in his book.[109] As noted earlier, in 1619, Van Otten described Atwood of Worcester, not Banister, as the best oculist in England.

In contrast with his uncle, Richard Banister continued to promulgate the incorrect idea that the lens is in "the middest of the eyes," which is perhaps not surprising, given that he cited Vesalius but not Colombo. We might be tempted to call Van Otten the grandfather of British ophthalmology, except that he was only 2 years older than Banister.

Banister believed that "old men see better with spectacles than young men."[110]

Banister's text incorporated the new term cataract: "Blood coming by the Nerves cause Pinnes, Webs, Spots, Cataracts, and Opilations."[111] Unlike Seabrooke, Banister defended bloodletting. Banister also used other harsh treatments, such as leeches. Banister wrote: "A golden needle is better for the Eyes, then a silver needle."[112] However, his will left to his son "my box of silver instruments."[113] Banister also noted: "Some put a lowse into the Eye" for treatment.[114] He clarified that the "lowse" was good for dry, dull, and obscure eyes, but not for inflamed eyes. Putting a louse in the eye was also advocated as far away as Alaska, by the native Kodiak.[115] Banister cautioned against "Licking the Eye with the Tongue," which is found in the traditional ophthalmology of both the Old and New Worlds. Banister recommended pterygium excision. Banister noted a number of problems that could occur with couching: release of a milky substance that appeared to have been contained in a "blather," that is, a bladder—the lens capsule. One could also experience hyphema, apparent subluxation of the cataract into the anterior chamber obscuring the uvea (iris); cataracts that were too soft to be displaced; movement of the cataract back into

---

106 James 2013, p. 57.

107 Banister 1971, np.

108 Banister 1971, np.

109 Leffler et al. "British Isles" 2021.

110 Banister 1971, np.

111 Banister 1971, np.

112 Banister 1971, np.

113 James 2013, p. 61.

114 Leffler et al. "British Isles" 2021.

115 Leffler et al. "British Isles" 2021.

the visual axis due to hardness of the cataract; and adherence of the cataract to the uvea (iris). He used the term "couched" and seems to be relating his own personal experiences. He described couching the cataract of a woman "in Walsingham in Norfolk," which was adherent to the uvea and required parting "many small threds, or rather haires" (synechiolysis). In the early postoperative period, she could not see well, but after some time, the vision improved, and his local reputation improved.[116] Banister cited Barrough's treatise. Unlike the "mountebankes," Banister insisted that the English oculists always couched cataracts indoors.[117]

Banister criticized the clinical outcomes of "strangers" (foreigners) who drew teeth while "on horsebacke." In 1616, Napier described Banister as an "Oculist." Banister reported curing of blindness, presumably by couching, 24 people in Norwich in 1609, and more in 1611, as certified by the mayor. Banister also visited London, Lincoln, and St. Edmundsbury. Banister noted that in 1 month in a distant city, he could see more blind patients than in 6 months in his own town.[118] Banister believed that performing a unilateral couching would prevent a cataract from developing in the other eye.[119] Banister noted that many were drinking substantial quantities of "Beere or Ale" in the morning to help their sight. He thought that excessive use of these drinks could actually impair vision, but accepted them in moderation.

Richard Banister's Breviary is known for being the first in the Western medical tradition to note the poor prognosis of couching the palpably hard eye. Banister did not actually use the term *glaucoma* in his Breviary, however. James wrote: "His remarks fell on stony ground and more than two hundred years were to pass before his teaching became part of the ophthalmic creed."[120] Perhaps, there was a delay of a century, but it seems that Banister's work enjoyed prolonged circulation and was ultimately influential. Banister was cited by English author William Drage in 1664, and also by Benedict Duddell in 1733. William Read republished an edited version of Banister's Breviary, along with the translation of Guillemeau, in 1706. Just 1 year later, in 1707, John Thomas Woolhouse wrote a letter describing angle-closure glaucoma, including the palpably hard eye with mydriasis, and called it *glaucome*. This was the first time the term *glaucoma* had been used to describe the palpably hard eye. From his lectures and letters, we know that Woolhouse was aware of Banister's work. Woolhouse's student Platner in 1745 also used the term *glaucoma* to describe the palpably hard eye with mydriasis. Demours, who wrote about the palpably hard eye with mydriasis in 1818, cited elsewhere both Woolhouse and Platner. Thus, the chain of citations from Banister in 1622 to Demours in 1818 demonstrates that Banister's work probably did have long-lasting influence.[121]

---

116 Leffler et al. "British Isles" 2021.

117 Leffler et al. "British Isles" 2021.

118 Leffler et al. "British Isles" 2021.

119 Leffler et al. "British Isles" 2021.

120 James 2013, p. 60.

121 Leffler et al. "British Isles" 2021; Leffler & Schwartz "Enlightenment" 2020, p. 199.

New Words: Cataract, Oculist, and Couching (by 1588)

It is only in the Elizabethan era that we have evidence of the terms "cataract," "couching," and "oculist" being applied to actual patients, procedures, or doctors in the British Isles. Both the early manuscript of Grassus' treatise and the later Middle English versions used the colloquial term "webbe" to describe a film on the eye.[122] Although the word *cataract* had been used in a Norman French manuscript, and in multiple Middle English manuscripts as early as 1380, the term *cataract* did not enter the English vernacular for another two centuries. Patients continued to be diagnosed as having a web, which was just a nonspecific term for an ocular media opacity or film, often on the cornea, but not necessarily. When Henry VIII authorized the use of herbalist remedies by unlicensed practitioners in 1543 (the so-called Quacks' Charter), he mentioned "a Pin and the Web in the Eye," but not cataract.[123]

The earliest use of the term "cataract" to describe an eye disease in an English patient was in a letter by the German doctor Valentine Russwurin in 1573 or 1574 when he briefly resided in London. John Banister noted in 1578 that some of the younger doctors were calling the disorder cataract. It is not until 1588 that we know of a native Englishman, physician Simon Forman, describing an English patient as having a "cataract."[124]

Likewise, the Middle English formulation of the Latin "oculistas" as "oculisterz" in the Chauliac manuscript of 1425 did not catch on. Ultimately, the Latin-derived word resurfaced in English as "oculist." The earliest known use in English was in 1588 when surgeon William Clowes listed a medical recipe: "This receit was giuen me for a secrete, of one I suppose to be a good occulist..."[125] The next known instance of a doctor in the British Isles being described as a "chirurgion and occulist" was Henry Blackborne in his certificate from the mayor of Rye of 1610 and then in his will of 1611. Physician and astrologer Richard Napier used the term "Oculist" to describe Richard Banister in 1616 and Atwood of Worcester in 1619.[126] Richard Seabrooke described himself as an "occulist" in his treatise of 1620.[127]

Roos' 1519 use of the term *couching* to describe cataract surgery is fascinating, because it comes so much earlier than any other instance. It is often noted that the English term *couching* is ultimately derived from the French verb *coucher*, meaning to lie down. Therefore, one might assume that the French used this verb to describe cataract surgery. But the French did not. For instance, Jacques Guillemeau discussed

---

122 Grassus 2011, pp. 500-501.

123 Leffler et al. "British Isles" 2021.

124 Leffler et al. "British Isles" 2021.

125 Leffler et al. "British Isles" 2021.

126 Leffler et al. "British Isles" 2021.

127 Seabrooke 1620, np.

which types of cataract were proper "à abbatre." Similarly, the Spanish referred to needles used to "abatir la catarata." This means "to bring down." It is true that in nonophthalmic contexts, the English word "couch" had been adapted from the French as early as the 14th century. But the use of the term *couch* to describe cataract surgery appears to be original in English. After 1519, the next known use of the term to describe cataract surgery was in 1587 with Anthony Hunton's translation of Guillemeau's treatise. Fenton's use in 1590 when translating Grassus' manuscript suggests that the term was becoming popular.[128]

Cataract Surgeons in Scotland (by 1595)

As with England, seemingly miraculous ophthalmic healings were performed by saints quite early in the Scottish medieval period. The introduction of couching into Scotland occurred several decades after its introduction into England. On February 5, 1588/1589, Philip Hislop, one of the regents of the college at Edinburgh, was granted a license to travel to London to seek care for an ophthalmic malady.[129] The Continental use of the term *cataract* for an eye disorder might have gained some popularity in Scotland in 1591 when King James VI (1566-1625) used the term in his translation of the poems of Guillaume de Salluste Du Bartas.[130]

The ability to perform cataract surgery may have arrived in Scotland in 1595. On August 1, 1595, in response to a complaint by local surgeons, a French surgeon, "Maister Awin [a] Parisian," was fined by the town council of Edinburgh for practicing despite not belonging to the guild. The council ordered that he restrict his practice to "the cutting of the stayne [lithotomy], the curing of that sort of rymbursin [hernia] quha hes their entrellis fallin in their bawcod [scrotum], the cataract or sluch of the eye, the pest and the diseases of wemin resultand upon their birth."[131]

Peter Lowe in Scotland (1598)

Surgeon Peter Lowe (c. 1550-1610) of Scotland trained and initially practiced in Paris. By early 1598, he was living in Glasgow. Lowe had some familiarity with cataract surgery from his time in France. Lowe had responded to one of his French professors: "...in blindness[s], the sight is abolished, dimished as suffocation as happeneth in the beginning of Catarack..."[132] Lowe also noted that one used "... in the eye, an instrume[n]t called speculu[m] oculi, a needle proper to abate the

---

128 Leffler et al. "British Isles" 2021.

129 Leffler et al. "British Isles" 2021. Some have written that King James IV of Scotland might have referred to, or even have performed himself, a cataract couching in 1501, because he gave money to a wife who "had hir eyne schorne." We have reviewed the question in detail and concluded that the woman could have just suffered an eye injury (Leffler et al. "British Isles" 2021).

130 Leffler et al. "British Isles" 2021.

131 Leffler et al. "British Isles" 2021.

132 Leffler et al. "British Isles" 2021.

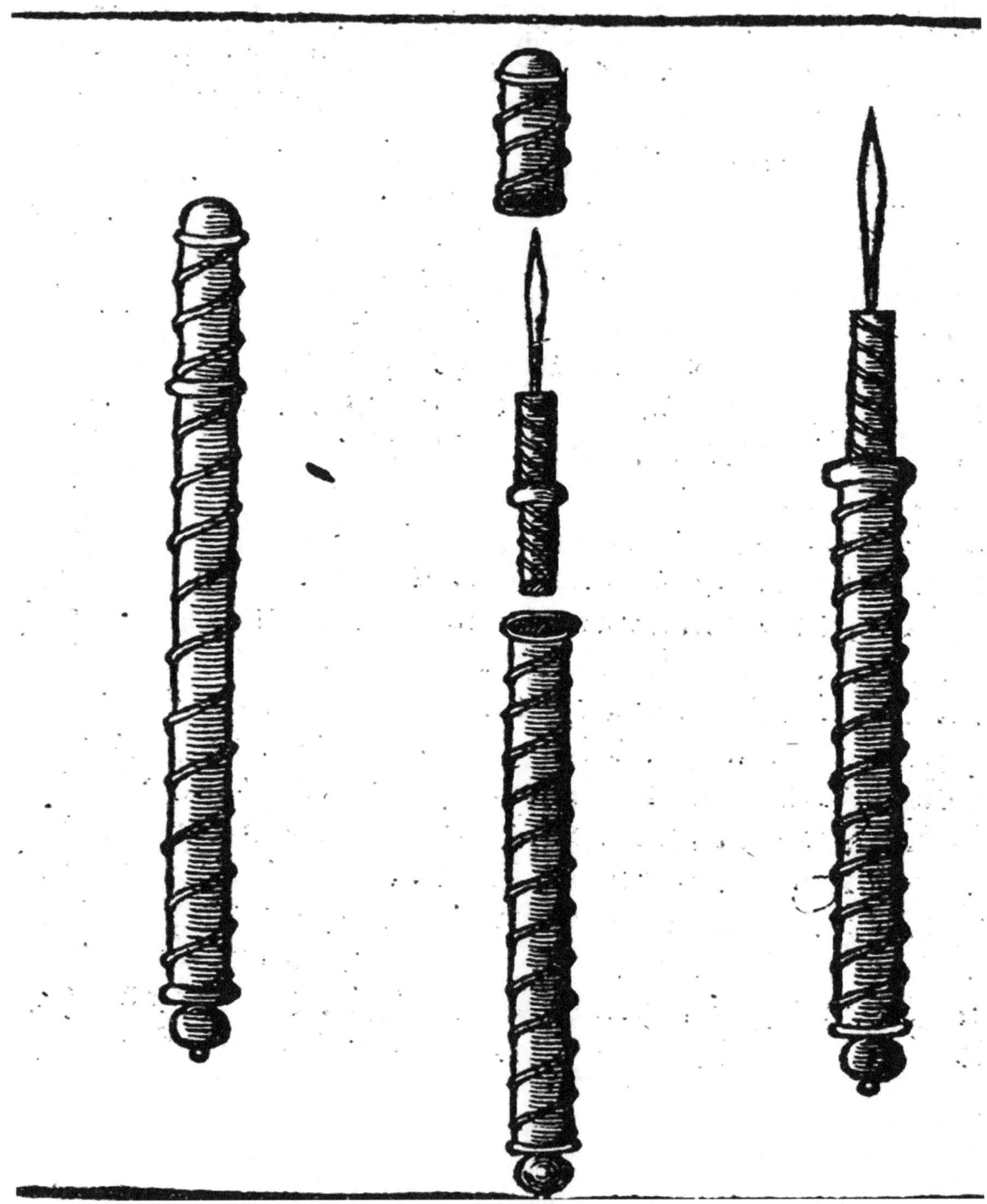

Fig. 6. Cataract couching needles from Peter Lowe's 1612 surgical treatise.

Cataract."[133] This was the anglicized version of the French verb *abattre*, rather than the English "to couch." The 1597 edition did not have a chapter explicitly discussing cataract surgery.[134]

The second edition of his surgical treatise was apparently printed posthumously in 1612 (Fig. 6). This second edition does have robust chapters on cataract diagnosis and surgery, and even uses the term "couching" to describe procedures that he personally performed. Lowe had a figure of a cataract needle that could be hidden in a protective metal covering. During the procedure, one would turn the needle "…until such time as you couch it to the lowest point of the eye…" He noted that in English the terms "cataract" and "tey" were synonymous. Lowe discussed the treatment of cataracts in several of his own patients.

As in England, there is little evidence that this introduction of cataract surgery really took root among academic or traditional surgeons. In 1627, Robert Archibald of Glasgow was admitted a freeman "in the calling of chirurgerie & in particular in the Incision of the Stone, Cataract, hernia…"[135] Archibald continues to be mentioned in the Faculty Minute books through 1641.

The competency examination by the Incorporation of Surgeons in Edinburgh of Andrew Johnston in 1712 did not mention cataracts, but that of James Robertson in 1719 included "couching of the cataract, fistula lachrimalis." Likewise, that of John Douglas in 1724 included "operation of couching the cataract, theory of vision."[136]

Echoes of Cataract Surgery in Shakespeare (1606)

William Shakespeare (1564-1616) wrote when cataract surgery was becoming widespread in England. It would not be surprising if this new procedure influenced his art, such as in King Lear, first performed in 1606. The Earl of Gloucester is blinded when Cornwall orders his servants "To this chaire bind him [Gloucester]" and gouges out Gloucester's eyes with his foot.[137] The image of a person tied to a chair and screaming as others damage their eyes would call to mind cataract surgery. Indeed, this procedure was sometimes performed in public on a stage.

In antiquity, the patient might be sitting close to the ground. However, by the medieval period, the patient was gradually elevated onto a bench and then a chair. According to the early 1400s Middle English translation of Grassus during the procedure, the surgeon should "…make the pacient to sitte on astole [a stool] and thou

---

133 Leffler et al. "British Isles" 2021.
134 Leffler et al. "British Isles" 2021.
135 Leffler et al. "British Isles" 2021.
136 Leffler et al. "British Isles" 2021.
137 Leffler et al. "British Isles" 2021. Act 3, Scene 7.

shalt sitte with the pacient face to face…"[138] A late 1400s manuscript was a little more clear that the patient and surgeon were facing each other while straddling the same bench as if riding a horse.[139] Lanfranc of Milan and Guy de Chauliac in 1363 also had the patient on a "stool" during the couching procedure. Chauliac had an attendant holding the patient's head still, while the patient's hands were placed under his own knees.[140]

Binding of the patient's limbs during cataract surgery had occurred at least since the 11th-century treatise of oculist 'Alī ibn 'Īsā al-Kahhal of Baghdad, known later in the west as Jesu Hali.[141] De Vigo in 1514 combined these ideas, as the patient was bound to a chair:

> comforte the patie[n]t, & set hym vpo[n] a streyght be[n]che of a meane height. Bynd the hole [nonoperative] eye, and also hys legges & hys ha[n]des, that he hynder not the operation of ye chirurgien.[142]

At the end of the attack in King Lear, Cornwall cries "out vild Ielly [vile jelly]," apparently referencing the vitreous. At a minimum, this line suggests that Shakespeare had some knowledge of the internal ocular structures. In 1594, Hester, a medical author, described how a splinter of wood impacted the eye of a maiden with such force that "the gellie of her eye came forth."[143] But Shakespeare may even have intended to suggest an eye disease. Many have seen parallels between the paradoxical themes in King Lear and in Charles Estienne's *Defence of Contraries*, translated in 1593, and have suggested that Shakespeare may have read this work.[144] In the chapter "That it is better to be blinde, then to see cleerely," Estienne refers to "eye-gellie" as an ophthalmic disease.[145] A 1611 translation from the French work of Du Bartas defined "catharact" as "a disease in the Eye distilling a tough humour like gelly."[146] In 1578, Thomas Cooper defined *cataracta* as "a disease of the eyes, when a tough humour like a gelly droppeth out."[147] This instance is particularly important because Shakespeare is thought to have used Cooper's dictionary.[148] Thus, if Shakespeare were intrigued by the new ophthalmic surgery sweeping the land, he might turn to a dictionary that compared a cataract to ocular jelly.

---

138 Grassus 2011, p. 227. Hunter MS 513.

139 (Grassus 2011, p. 224. Hunter MS 503. In the Latin treatises of Grassus published in 1474, the word used for seat was "sedere," as it was in other Latin manuscripts (Grassus 2011, p. 224).

140 Leffler et al. "British Isles" 2021.

141 Leffler et al. "Annals" 2020.

142 Leffler et al. "British Isles" 2021.

143 Leffler et al. "British Isles" 2021.

144 Leffler et al. "British Isles" 2021.

145 Leffler et al. "British Isles" 2021.

146 Leffler et al. "British Isles" 2021.

147 Leffler et al. "British Isles" 2021.

148 Leffler et al. "British Isles" 2021.

The Mountebanks (by the 1630s)

In the 17th century, the family continued to be an important vehicle for transmitting ophthalmic knowledge, but another institution also served this purpose: mountebank troupes. Sometimes, these institutions overlapped, when the troupes were family affairs. Universities and hospitals were not the prominent teachers of cataract surgery in this era.

Mountebanks had probably been present in the British Isles for many years. In 1622, Banister derided "quacksalving Mountebankes" who performed their cures outdoors at markets, sometimes on scaffolds, after playing a trumpet.[149]

One accusation against itinerants is that they might move on before the postoperative recovery was complete. Banister remembered that Blackborne's former student Hanle "would neuer stay in a place where he had couched Cataracts, till their eyes were opened but traueled in haste..."[150] Physician James Primerose (c. 1598-1659) in a diatribe against mountebanks, actually approved of itinerant cataract surgeons.[151]

Beginning in the 1630s, mountebanks operated on a grander scale in the British Isles. This trend began with John Ponteus, thought to be of Italy, who had traveled to London with a 10-person troupe by 1630.[152] Ponteus was described by physician Walter Harris in 1683 as "Pontaeus, the first Mountebank that ever appeared on a Stage in England."[153] The entertainment provided by Ponteus consisted of "stage playis" by 1643, and by 1663, both rope dancing, and sliding on a taut rope "his hands low and streatched out lyke the winges of a fowel."[154] Ponteus took his entourage to Oxford University and traveled throughout England and Scotland. Another prominent mountebank was Salvator Winter. The lay publications of both Ponteus and Winter emphasized medicines. However, Ponteus was licensed to practice surgery and published works on surgery. Winter called himself "an expert operator" and offered "to Cut, and Cure" a number of ailments.[155] Moreover, subsequent cataract couchers, such as John Church and William Read, cited Ponteus and Winter as authorities. Church claimed to have trained with them. Read called Ponteus his master and lauded Winter's medical formulas. Therefore, at a minimum, Ponteus and Winter inspired subsequent generations of oculists.

In addition to medical care, the mountebanks provided entertainment. Edward Green, the younger (d. 1745), had rope dancers and tumblers perform on a stage

---

149 Leffler et al. "British Isles" 2021.
150 Leffler et al. "British Isles" 2021.
151 Leffler et al. "British Isles" 2021.
152 Leffler et al. "British Isles" 2021.
153 Leffler et al. "British Isles" 2021.
154 Leffler et al. "British Isles" 2021.
155 Leffler et al. "British Isles" 2021.

in Edinburgh. The audience was asked to throw a handkerchief containing one or two shillings, and the handkerchief would generally be returned with medicine. Sometimes, a silver cup might be returned in the handkerchief, to encourage the patients to gamble.[156]

Usually, the entertainment took a back seat to the performance of surgery and the sale of medicines. But in one family, dancing and acrobatics were the main attractions. Andreas Larini (also known as Signor Violante), the husband of a professional dancer, performed acrobatic feats of rope sliding. He slid down a rope on May 31, 1727, from the steeple of St. Martin-in-the-Fields, Westminster, and in July 1728, slid across the River Severn, while firing a pistol held in each hand. Violante has been identified as one of the acrobats on the ropes in Hogarth's painting "Southwark Fair" of 1733. Thereafter, the Signor adopted a less adventuresome career. He advertised as "Andreas Laurini," a long-time "occulist" in Dublin in May 1731 when his wife performed there. In 1735, "Mr. Larini" danced with his wife in the Newcastle theater.[157]

Not only did the mountebanks conduct a large portion of the eye surgeries, but their troupes also functioned as educational institutions. Sometimes, as in the case of the Green family, these mountebanks were training their own kinsmen. But in many cases, the knowledge was transmitted to apprentices who were hired. There are stories of apprentices running away, with advertisements declaring them imposters or seeking their apprehension. In 1724, oculist Roger Grant advertised that William Grant was his footman and, despite William's claims, had never been instructed "in the Ophthalmic Art."[158] William Grant retorted that he had indeed learned couching from his Uncle Roger. William Grant (d. 1769) went on to have a long career in Reading.[159]

In 1793, John Dunn, an apprentice to the Liverpool oculist Mr. Johnson, ran away. A one guinea reward was posted for the apprehension and delivery of Dunn to a druggist. Dunn escaped and was advertising as "Dr. Dunn, Occulist" from 1799 to 1826.[160]

Despite the possibility of learning a trade, working as an assistant could be exploitive and even dangerous. Walter Harris (1647-1732) heard that Ponteus "made a Challenge to the Physicians at Oxford, to prepare for one of his Servants, the Rankest Poyson that they could contrive."[161] According to Harris, the servant survived the poison by eating several pounds of butter in advance to coat his stomach

---

156 Leffler et al. "British Isles" 2021.

157 Leffler et al. "British Isles" 2021.

158 Leffler et al. "British Isles" 2021.

159 Leffler et al. "British Isles" 2021.

160 Leffler et al. "British Isles" 2021.

161 Leffler et al. "British Isles" 2021.

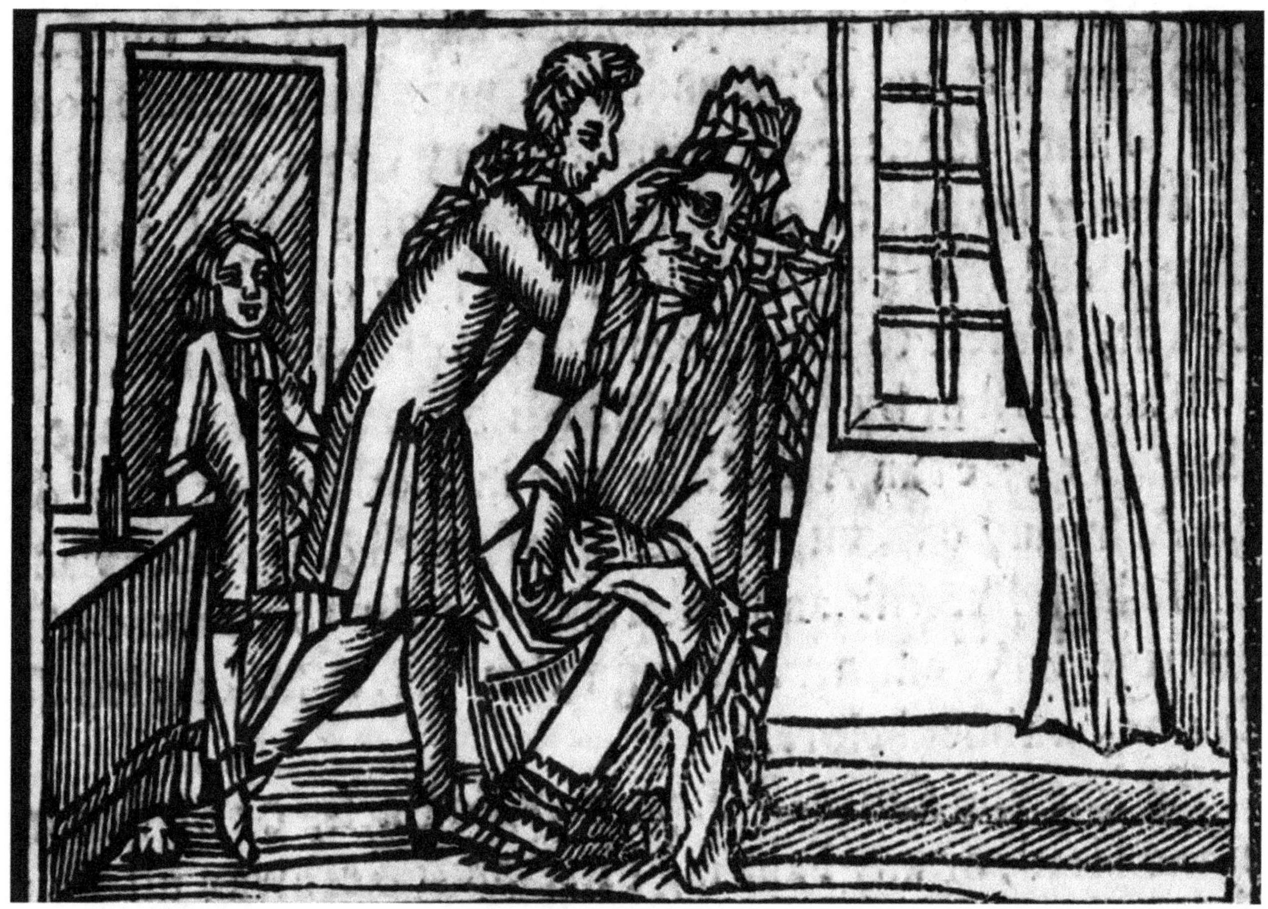

Fig. 7. A handbill of Cornelius Tilborg from the time of King William III (1694–1702) showing the doctor couching a cataract.

and then, after collapsing on stage and being removed from site, vomiting up the poison. Thus, it seems the Oxford physicians were complicit in the whole episode.

In 1684, the mountebank Cornelius Tilborg erected a stage in Edinburgh and attempted to prove the efficacy of his antidotes after one of his servants ingested poison. However, the experiment failed, and the servant died.[162] A handbill of Cornelius Tilborg from the time of King William III (1694–1702) features an illustration of Tilborg apparently couching a cataract (Fig. 7).[163]

In 1695, Edward Green (d. 1729) complained to the Justices of the Peace in Middlesex that his apprenticeship to Roger Gateley did not involve surgical instruction. Rather, Gateley "compelled him to practice the art and employment of rope-dancing, tumbling, and acting as a jack-pudding, on a mountebank's stage…and… Gateley also had at several times immoderately beat and misused his said apprentice."[164]

---

162 Leffler et al. "British Isles" 2021.

163 Mullini 2016, p. 119.

164 Leffler et al. "British Isles" 2021.

The Justices permitted Green to be relieved of his obligations as an apprentice. Green went on to have a successful career as the patriarch of three generations of itinerant oculists.

Harris heard that Ponteus would have an assistant howl in pain when what looked like molten lead was poured over his hands, only to be miraculously healed by an ointment. The secret was that the apparent lead was really "Quick-silver" (mercury).[165]

In 1687, an oculist named "Doctor Reid" (possibly Richard Reidman) in Edinburgh filed litigation against a couple "for stealing away from him a little girl called the Tumbling Lassie, who danced upon his stage; she danced in all shapes, and, to make her supple, he daily oiled all her joints…he had bought her from her mother for £30 Scots."[166] However, physicians testified that "the employment of tumbling would bruise all her bowels and kill her; and her joints were now grown stiff."[167] The mountebank lost his case.

Traditional ophthalmic histories downplay the importance of the mountebank in the latter half of the 17th century by emphasizing the practice of Daubeney Turberville (c. 1612-1696) of Salisbury. He was well connected to the country's elite political and academic circles and attended Oxford University from 1634 to 1640. Some university historians have implied that he learned ophthalmology at Oxford. In fact, we do not know where Turberville learned to practice as an oculist, but it could very well have been through family connections or from the mountebanks who visited Oxford. It is not clear that any of the doctors at Oxford during Turberville's time there knew how to couch cataracts. According to Pope, Turberville "bore Arms for the King" during the English Civil War.[168] He is probably the "chirurgeon or oculist" who spied for the royal side in January 1645/1646, acting as an agent of Lord George Digby (1612–1677), the second Earl of Bristol, who also attended Oxford.[169] During the rule of Oliver Cromwell, Turberville was relegated to be a provincial oculist in the 1650s in Crookhorn. He was almost certainly the oculist from "Crewkerne" who was paid 3 pounds by the town of Dorchester to perform cataract surgeries on an older couple. With the restoration of the monarchy in 1660, Turberville was now rewarded for his previous royal support. He was awarded an essentially honorary MD degree at Oxford and traveled to London to provide medical care to elites, such as Samuel Pepys and Princess Anne. He resided in Salisbury, where one could see an abundance of his patients being led by boys or women, with a bandage over one or both eyes, or green silk covering their face, according to Pope. However, Turberville's training appears to have been empiric, rather than academic. It was not until 1668 that, while at an alehouse with friends, he had the opportunity to observe the

---

165 Leffler et al. "British Isles" 2021.
166 Leffler et al. "British Isles" 2021.
167 Leffler et al. "British Isles" 2021.
168 Leffler et al. "British Isles" 2021.
169 Leffler et al. "British Isles" 2021.

dissection of an eye. Pepys was incredulous that such a famous oculist would not have previously seen the interior of the eye. Turberville was said to have learned how to perform paracentesis to release aqueous from a ship captain who had spent 15 years in Peking. Turberville may have also had connections with the Stepkins–Woolhouse dynasty of oculists, given that he was said to have demonstrated paracentesis for Thomas Woolhouse. Paracentesis for a new condition called hydrophthalmia was just entering Europe at the end of the 17th century, as oculists were inspired by the Asian practice of acupuncture.[170]

Honoratus Le Begg received a medical license in 1668 from the diocese of Canterbury and was still active in 1677. He then disappeared until 1694, when he advertised in London that "Doctor Lebeg, Oculist…eminent for Couching of Cataracts" was traveling to Spain to treat an eminent blind person with cataracts when he was captured by a "Turks Man of War," sold as a slave in Algiers and then Egypt, where he remained for 2 years before returning to practice in the North of England.[171]

The most prominent eye surgeon in the British Isles in the decades following Turberville was William Read, of England. Historians have differed radically in their assessment of Read. His Oxford biographer wrote: "Sir William was a more effective self-promoter and plagiarist than he was an oculist."[172] However, we agree more with the historian who wrote that Read was the "best eye man in England."[173] In order to understand Read, it is essential to study the progression in his career. Read probably began working in the medical field in some capacity by about 1673. Both antiquarian Le Neve and Read himself, probably in about 1691, indicated that Read got his start working under John Ponteus. Ponteus had faded from the scene by about 1676, but perhaps the careers of Ponteus and Read overlapped by a few years. In any event, Read saw himself in his early days as carrying on the tradition of one of the most theatrical mountebanks in the British Isles, a man who was accused of using deception in his stage shows. It was probably in about 1691 when Read published "a catalogue of those medicaments he sold off his stages during the time of his eighteen years travelling in England, Scotland, Ireland, and many foreign kingdoms."[174]

But Read evolved. His first gambit was to take his stage presentations to the major universities (Fig. 8).[175] In 1684, he couched cataracts in Dublin and received a certificate from officials at Trinity College. In 1689, he treated patients at Oxford University, reportedly to the satisfaction of the spectators. In 1697, he treated patients at Cambridge University. Although Read performed surgeries and probably sold medicines from his stage, there is no evidence he performed plays, hired

---

170 Leffler & Schwartz "Woolhouse" 2017.

171 Leffler et al. "British Isles" 2021.

172 Leffler et al. "British Isles" 2021.

173 Leffler et al. "British Isles" 2021.

174 Leffler et al. "British Isles" 2021.

175 James 2013, pp. 126-9.

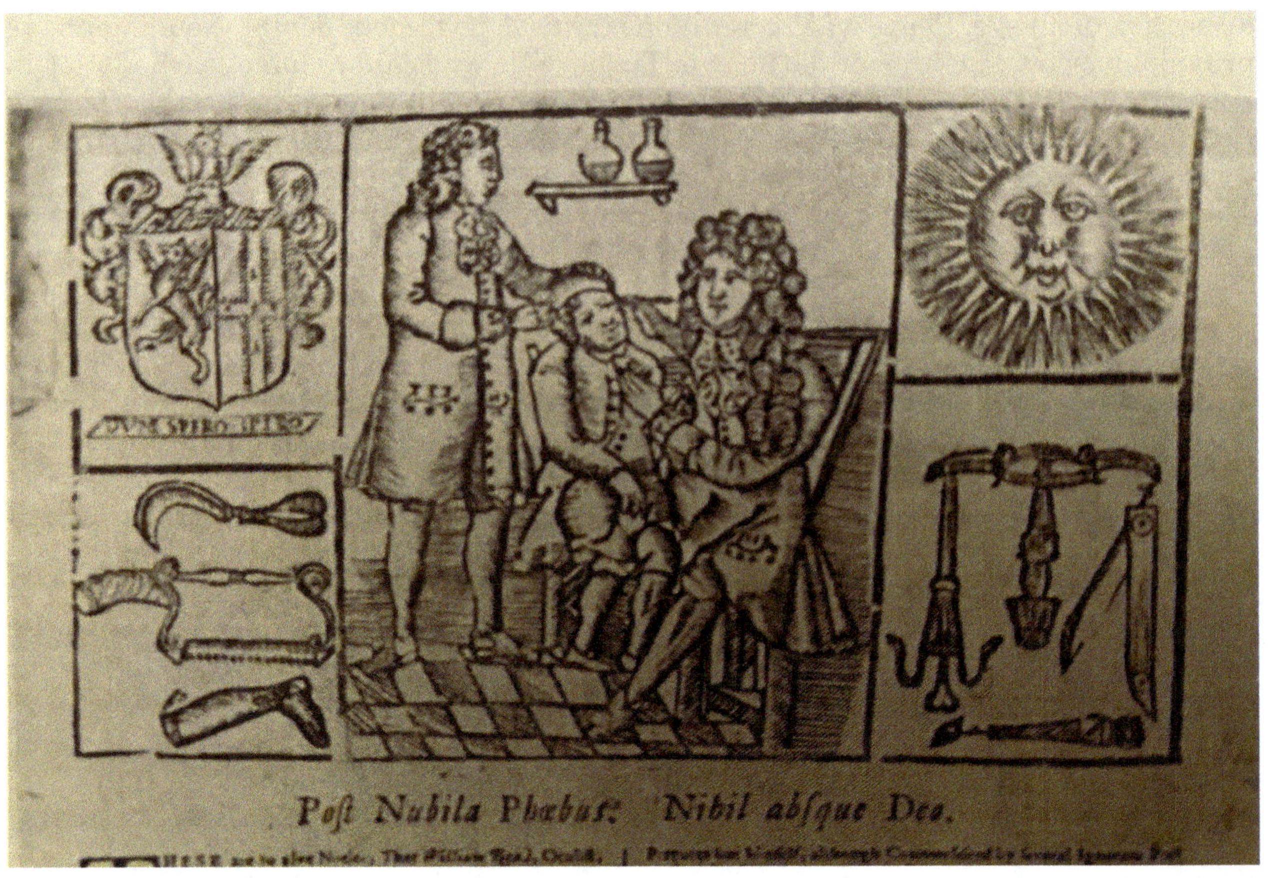

Fig. 8. William Read's handbill of 1694 from the British Library shows him couching a man indoors.

dancers, or had assistants poisoned or bitten by snakes. Perhaps, in his early days as a junior servant to Ponteus or others, Read engaged in such theatrics (we have no way of knowing), but when on his own, he chose not to do so. When Jonathan Swift received an invitation to a party from Read, Swift wrote that Read "has been a mountebank," not that he still was one.[176]

Read's success at the universities led to opportunities to treat the ruling class. Read was the dominant oculist in London during the period, which saw the couching of physician Peter Barwick (1619-1705) in 1692 and of Lady Rachel Russell (1637-1723) in 1694 and 1695. As an oculist, Read became in 1698 the "Servant in Ordinary to His present Majesty" (King William III). In 1702, Read couched the cataract of Sir Cecil Bishopp, fourth Baronet (c. 1635-1705). In August 1705, Read was knighted by Queen Anne for the charity care he provided to soldiers and sailors. Read was recommended as the best surgeon for couching cataracts by William Coward in his *Ophthalmiatria* of 1706. Read's couching of the cataract of parliamentarian Simon

---

176 Leffler et al. "British Isles" 2021.

Harcourt (1661-1727) in August 1710 was successful and was followed by Harcourt's reappointment as attorney general the following month.[177]

From the mid-1690s onward, Read was no longer a mountebank performing on a stage. He advertised in newspapers that patients could come to his house to be treated. He still practiced as an itinerant throughout England. In his absence, he would leave first his brother-in-law the oculist J. Brinsden in London to treat his patients, beginning in 1703, and then, beginning in 1709, his wife Augustina, the Lady Read.[178] Both of these family members couched cataracts. For most of the oculists of this period, we have very little outcomes data, independent of the oculist's own advertisements. Unfavorable outcomes might occasionally be publicized by a competitor, but we could not find such reports with respect to Read. Couching in this era undoubtedly could fail frequently, but given his high surgical volume and the ability to readily find patients at all strata of society, we might imagine that his outcomes were as good as anyone else's.

His critics have focused not on his outcomes, but on the oxymoronic charge that he was an illiterate plagiarist. Given that Read published Banister's work, incorporating his own edits, and that there is a manuscript in Read's own hand, it seems that he could read and write English.[179] The charge of illiteracy is best interpreted to mean that he lacked formal university education and could not read Latin or Greek well. Another criticism of Read in the modern day, and in one letter of the period by Woolhouse, is that Read plagiarized Banister's 1622 treatise. In fact, neither Banister nor Read acknowledged Guillemeau as the original source. What both authors did was quite similar. Both put their names on a volume that contained the material of others, to which each added his own section (Banister's Breviary and Read's Practical Observations). Defenders of Banister and Read could argue that they put their own name on the section they wrote but not at the start of the sections borrowed from predecessors. The standards of the period were still evolving, and this type of copying without attribution was quite common. We cannot lionize Banister as the heroic and unblemished father of British ophthalmology while condemning Read as a mountebank and plagiarist. Both were itinerants who read and republished ophthalmic works in English (without explicit acknowledgment of the source), while adding their own unique observations. Upon Read's death in 1715, his wife carried on the practice.[180]

One of the most prominent itinerant oculists of the 18th century in the British Isles, and all of Europe, was John Taylor. He had experience with scholarly, hospital-based surgeons and with an itinerant oculist and fused the academic lecture with the stage presentation of the mountebank. Rather than traditional entertainment, such as acrobats, he presented a scholarly lecture, oriented toward laypeople,

---

177 Leffler et al. "British Isles" 2021.

178 James 2013, p. 125.

179 Read 1709.

180 Leffler et al. "British Isles" 2021.

community surgeons, and university doctors. Hans-Reinhard Koch has noted that Taylor might have inspired Jacques Daviel to practice as an itinerant oculist during Taylor's visit to Marseille in 1734.[181] In fact, Taylor might have also inspired William Cheselden to pursue ophthalmology in a public manner. We have no evidence that Cheselden performed eye surgery before Taylor spent time training under him at St. Thomas's Hospital. As Cheselden was an established surgeon, Taylor benefited by touting his time with Cheselden at the beginning of Taylor's ophthalmic treatise of 1727. Still, Taylor seemed to damn Cheselden with faint praise by noting "the little Damage you have ever done, where Unavoidable Accidents have conspir'd to render the Operation unsuccesful, is a great Evidence of the Accuracy of your Judgment."[182] Taylor's grandson suggested that the training with Cheselden was of a general nature. Taylor touted his success performing cataract surgeries in his hometown of Norwich in July 1726 before newspaper notices regarding Cheselden's cataract surgeries began appearing in March 1727. Likewise, Taylor's first ophthalmic treatise in 1727 preceded the first scholarly ophthalmic publications by Cheselden in 1728. Taylor did not find his ophthalmic training at St. Thomas's Hospital to be adequate. Thus, he spent 1729 touring Edinburgh and the rest of Scotland, apparently with an oculist who engaged in a "Method of public Practice."[183] We would note that the timing is consistent with the Scottish travels of Edward Green, the younger (d. 1745).

Taylor was actually well versed in the scholarship of the day. He was the first to draw the semi-decussation of the optic nerves.[184] He gave an excellent description of angle-closure glaucoma. Taylor was taken seriously by many of the established oculists and professors of the period. Thomas Hope had studied in Paris under Charles de St. Yves and John Thomas Woolhouse and still felt it worth his while to spend 6 months with Taylor in Edinburgh in 1743. On the other hand, in 1744, the Royal College of Physicians and the Corporation of Surgeons in Edinburgh cautioned against accepting Taylor's claims and warned that some of his surgeries were unsuccessful. Taylor was accused by Le Cat of pretending to perform strabismus surgery by operating on the deviating eye, patching the sound eye, and declaring success when the strabismic eye was used to fixate. We previously noted a newspaper report that confirmed that an oculist was conducting this charade in England in about 1742.[185] Our present efforts have provided the perspective that other English oculists were not trying to treat strabismus during this period. Thus, this oculist was most likely Taylor, and Le Cat's story is confirmed.

Taylor went on to become one of the most prominent oculists in all of Europe. His many accomplishments must be balanced against his flamboyance (he called himself "Chevalier") and his self-aggrandizement, which was deemed excessive

---

181 Leffler et al. "British Isles" 2021
182 Leffler et al. "British Isles" 2021.
183 Leffler et al. "British Isles" 2021.
184 Schwartz & Leffler "Taylor" 2020.
185 Schwartz & Leffler "Taylor" 2020.

even by the standards of his day. In addition, he had many unsatisfied patients, particularly on the Continent. He was forced to refund surgical fees in Mannheim, sued for malpractice in multiple locations, and forbidden to perform eye surgery in Habsburg territories. One might be tempted to say that Taylor's legacy lies in the work of his son and grandsons, who practiced as oculists in London. However, their style was that of the conventional oculist planting roots in one community. One who modeled himself on Taylor more completely was James Graham, who toured early America as an oculist, and adopted Taylor's slogans and style as an itinerant oculist presenting academic lectures.[186]

Female Oculists (by 1649)

Women have long played a role in providing medical care, learning within the family or from other women. However, their role was often unofficial. Surviving records do not list any female physicians in the time of King Henry (c. 1100). Given their central role in family life, it is not surprising that there is a long history of women providing medical care, even as early as the medieval period. The wife of a medieval doctor or barber would sometimes help in his practice, and even take over his practice upon his death.

Richard Banister derided women practitioners: "Let these women therefore either applie themselves to learne the grounds of their practice, or leave their practice to them that are better grounded; that so they may cease by their ignorance to make them blinde, that by our Arte might be made to see." Banister had no objection to a few women practitioners who worked "for charity" and presumably did not compete with him for the paying patients.[187]

When cataract surgery moved into the British Isles, this new procedure became integrated into the life of medical families. There was a brief period when women not only provided medical care, but even performed intraocular surgeries.

An interesting procedure was related by physician Theodore Mayerne (1573-1655), who arrived in England by 1611 and retired by 1649. A female English oculist (*Mulier Angla oculista*) drained the aqueous humor (*humorem Aqueum*), which had grown muddy and opaque (*turbidus & obscurior*), by inserting a needle into the cornea.[188] The eye collapsed but was restored when the aqueous was replenished, and the vision returned. If the aqueous that was drained had been clear, this case would upset our understanding of ophthalmic history, given that we do not know of paracentesis for hydrophthalmia being performed in Europe until the 1680s, when acupuncture was imported from Asia.[189] However, drainage of hypopyon, as in this case, had long been practiced in Europe. The patient was described as My Lord Rich,

---

186 Leffler et al. "British Isles" 2021.
187 Banister 1971, np.
188 Leffler et al. "British Isles" 2021.
189 Leffler & Schwartz "Woolhouse" 2017.

son of the Earl of Warwick, that is, Robert Rich (1611-1659). Our patient was known to have traveled to the Isle of Wight in July 1648 to be touched for "the king's evil" (tuberculosis). Parliamentarian intelligence suspected that this diagnosis was an excuse to visit the king, but all agreed he had some sort of illness: "The Lord Rich [eldest son of the earl of Warwick] is with the King. The pretence is to be touched for the King's Evil, his disease being another."[190] Thus, the hypopyon drainage could have been performed in the setting of uveitis, possibly from tuberculosis.

The oculist draining the hypopyon could have been any number of women. Lady Katherine Partridge Springett (1599-1647) of Kent was known for "taking off cataracts and spots in eyes," and was a colleague of John Stepkins (d. 1652).[191] Stepkins' daughter Lady Ivy was also known as an oculist. By 1655, Robert Boyle knew of an oculist named Mrs. Hunt. Mary Rich (1625-1678), the sister of Robert Boyle and sister-in-law of our patient, was known for "Chirurgery and Physick," as were several of her female colleagues.[192]

Some decades later, we learn of female oculists performing cataract surgery. Daubeney Turberville's sister, Mary Turberville, practiced after his death in 1696. Likewise, William Read's wife, Augustina, was couching cataracts by 1709.[193]

The poet William Cowper (1731-1800) had "specks" on his eyes and, therefore, was sent at age 8 to live with "Mrs. D, an eminent oculist." We believe that this was the oculist Mrs. Frances Deane, who learned from Mrs. Jones (d. 1720) and had died by 1754.[194]

One pattern observed is that women did not learn medicine from men outside their family. The only exception we encountered was a 14-year-old named Charles Hamilton, who apprenticed in 1740 with the oculist Edward Green (the younger, d. 1745), and then Finly Green, before practicing independently. After marrying a woman in 1746, Hamilton was discovered to be a woman named Mary who had impersonated a man. Hamilton was convicted of fraud and sentenced to be whipped.[195]

Surgical Illustrations (1674)

It is not until the age of the itinerants of the last quarter of the 16th century that we have surviving illustrations of couching needles in the British Isles. Peter Lowe included figures of couching needles in his surgical treatises of 1597 and 1612. Eye instruments, including couching needles, were also drawn in the 1598 translation

---

190 Leffler et al. "British Isles" 2021.

191 Leffler et al. "Stepkins" 2014.

192 Leffler et al. "British Isles" 2021.

193 Leffler et al. "British Isles" 2021.

194 Subsequent biographers have erroneously written that this was one "Mrs. Disney," but there is no evidence of an oculist named Disney (Leffler et al. "British Isles" 2021).

195 Leffler et al. "British Isles" 2021.

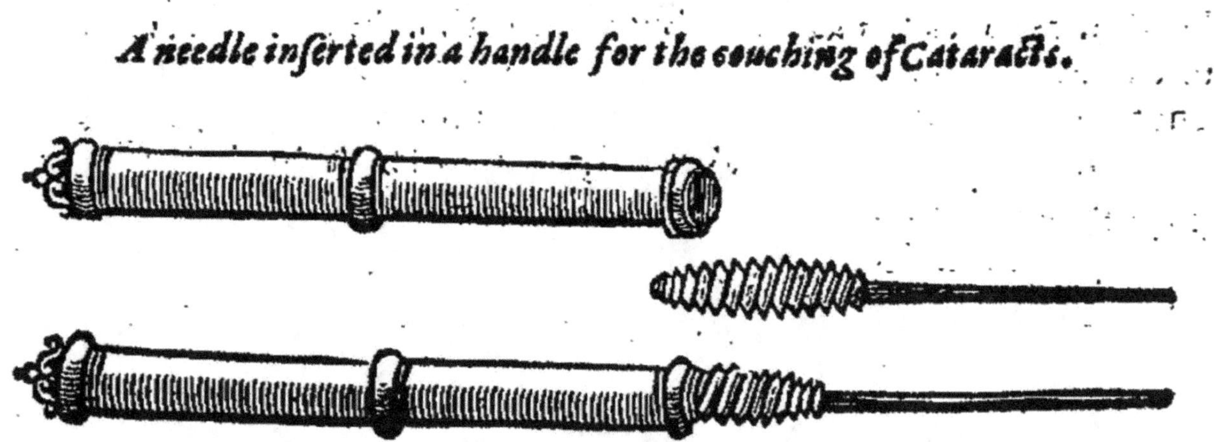

Fig. 9. Couching needle with handle from 1634 translation of Ambroise Paré's treatise.

of Jacques Guillemeau's *The Frenche chirurgerye*. The 1634 translation of Ambroise Paré's works also depicted a cataract couching needle, which screwed into a handle (Fig. 9).

On the continent, illustrations of cataract couching can be found from the early 16th century (Fig. 10). It is well into the 17th century that we begin to find surviving illustrations of cataract surgery from the British Isles. In the 1674 translation of the surgical treatise of Johannes Scultetus of Germany, we find drawings of "silver needles fit to couch a cataract." Scultetus also depicted the head of a patient with "a suffusion in the right eye, that…must be put down with a needle…"[196] It was actually the patient's left eye being couched with the doctor's right hand, and the nonsurgical eye was covered with a cloth (Figs. 11 and 12).

The first illustration of a couching procedure drawn by an Englishman might be that of John Browne (1642-c. 1700) in his 1678 treatise (Fig. 13). No cover can be seen over the nonoperative eye, even though the accompanying text recommended the surgeon "bind up the contrary Eye." Browne's treatise was later criticized by John Yonge (1647-1721). Yonge specifically noted that the cataract surgery illustration did not have "the other eye bound fast."[197] Yonge's general criticism of Browne was for plagiarism and incompleteness, but Yonge did not accuse Browne of copying the illustration.

John Russell's handbills illustrated the "couching a cataract of one that had been blind 30 years" (Fig. 14). A man with his sound (right) eye covered with a cloth gazes straight forward as the couching needle enters the temporal aspect of his left eye. Bibliographers have guessed that this handbill might date from 1680, but given

---

196 Leffler et al. "British Isles" 2021.
197 Leffler et al. "British Isles" 2021.

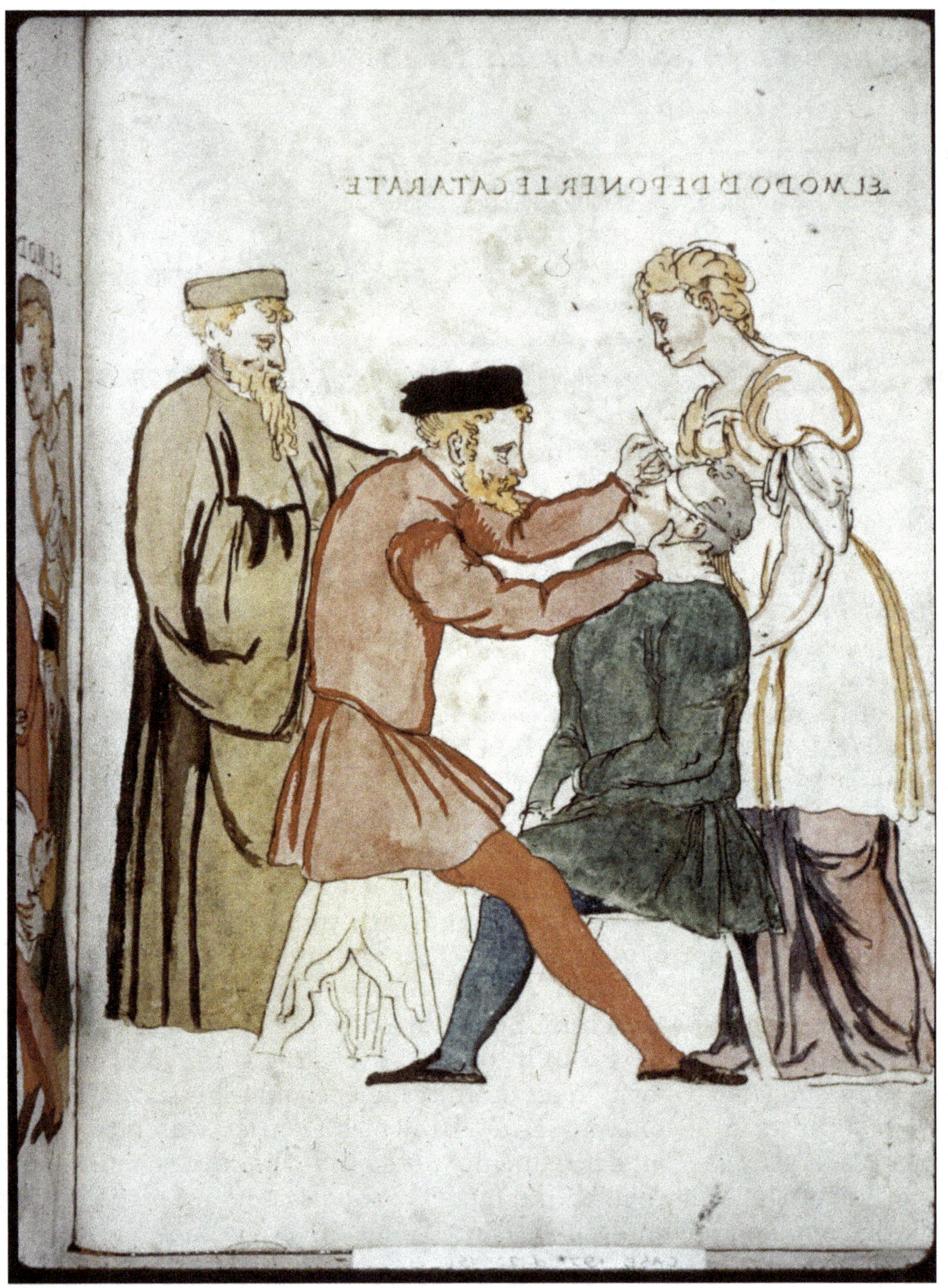

Fig. 10. An illustration of cataract couching from an Italian medical manuscript of 1510 by Henricus Kullmaurer and Albert Meher. The attendant is a woman.

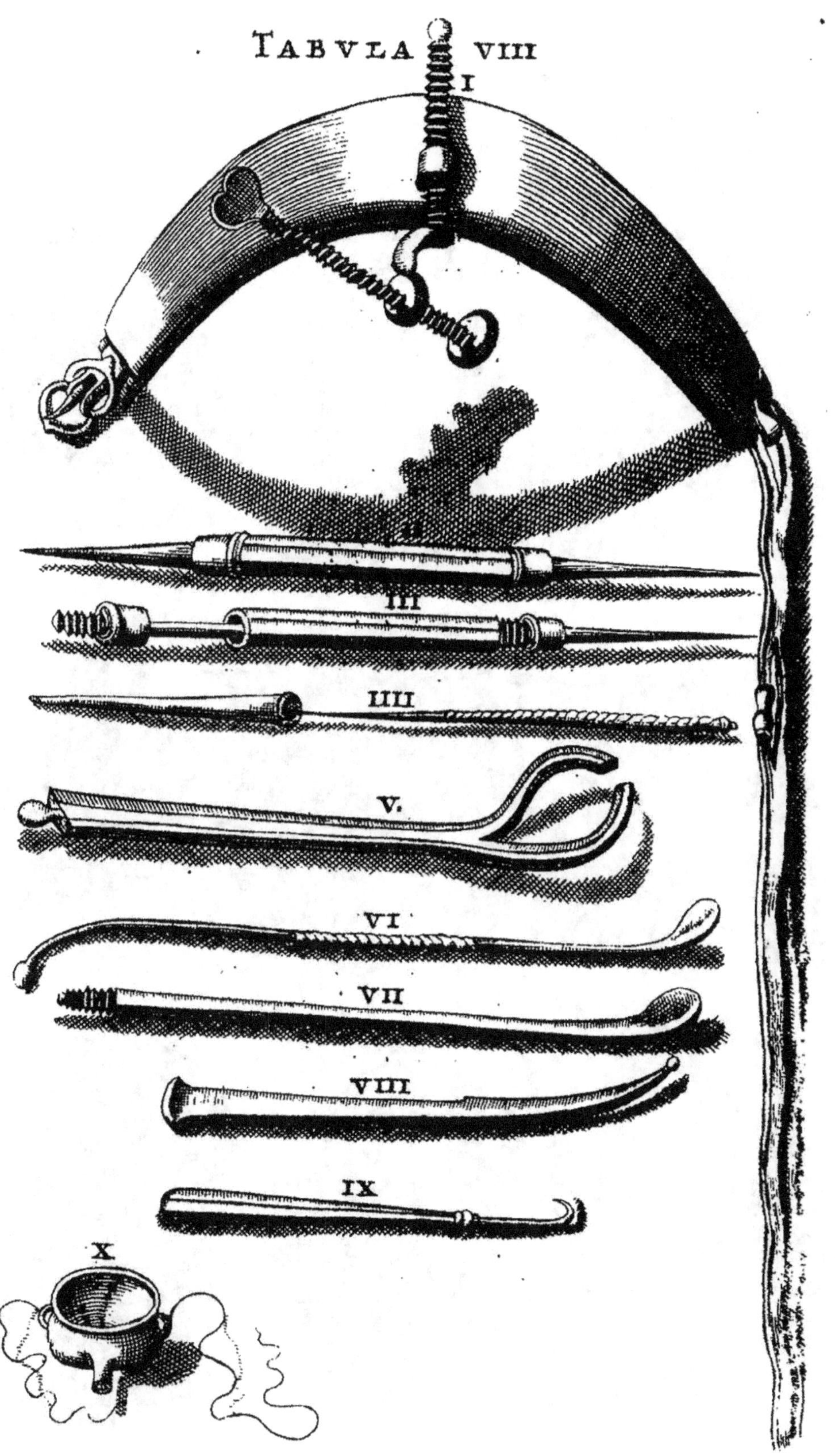

Fig. 11. Ophthalmic instruments, including silver couching needles, from the 1674 translation of the surgical treatise of Johannes Scultetus.

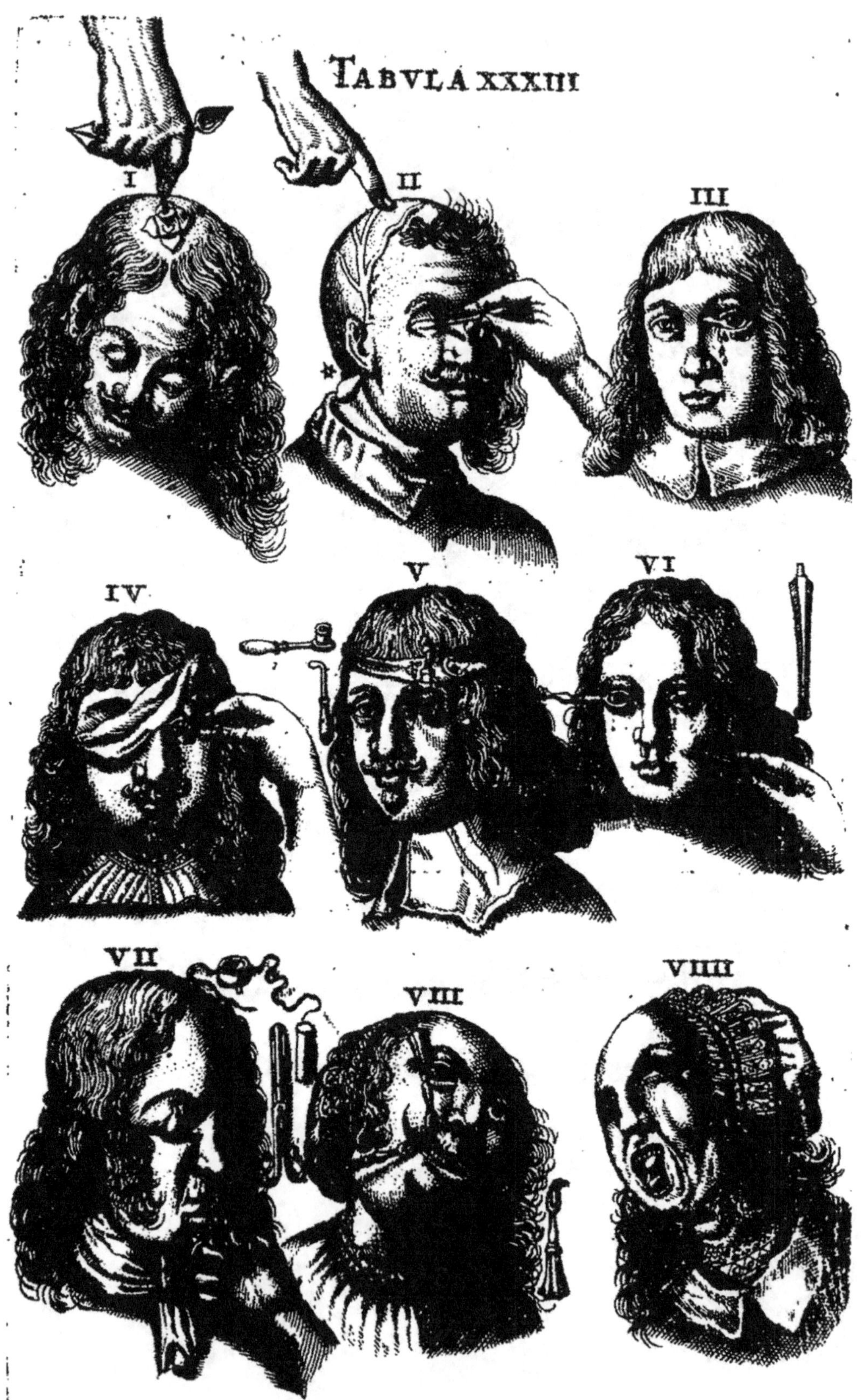

Fig. 12. Surgical procedures, including cataract couching (panel IV), from the 1674 translation of the surgical treatise of Johannes Scultetus.

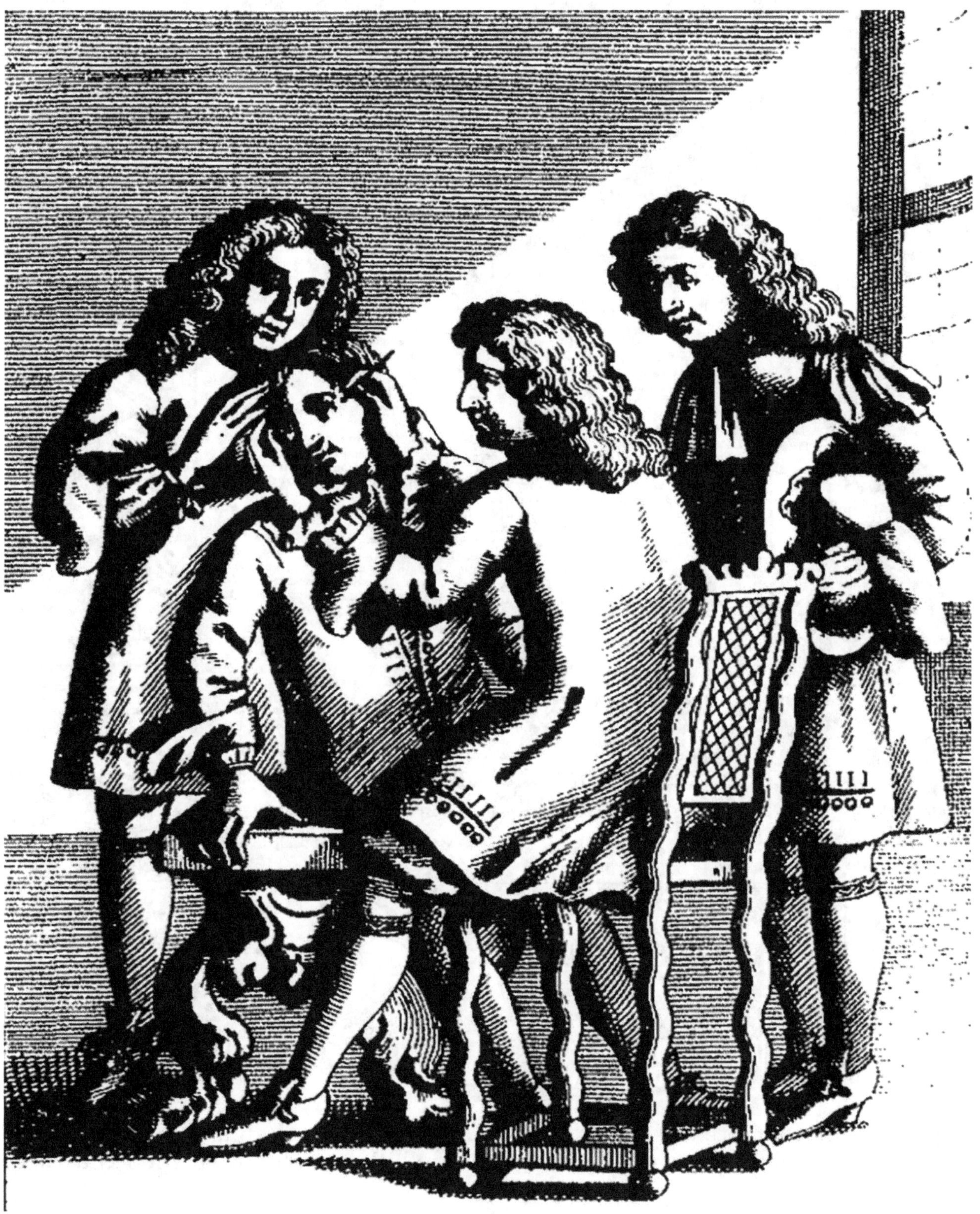

Fig. 13. Cataract couching illustration in the 1678 surgical treatise of John Browne.

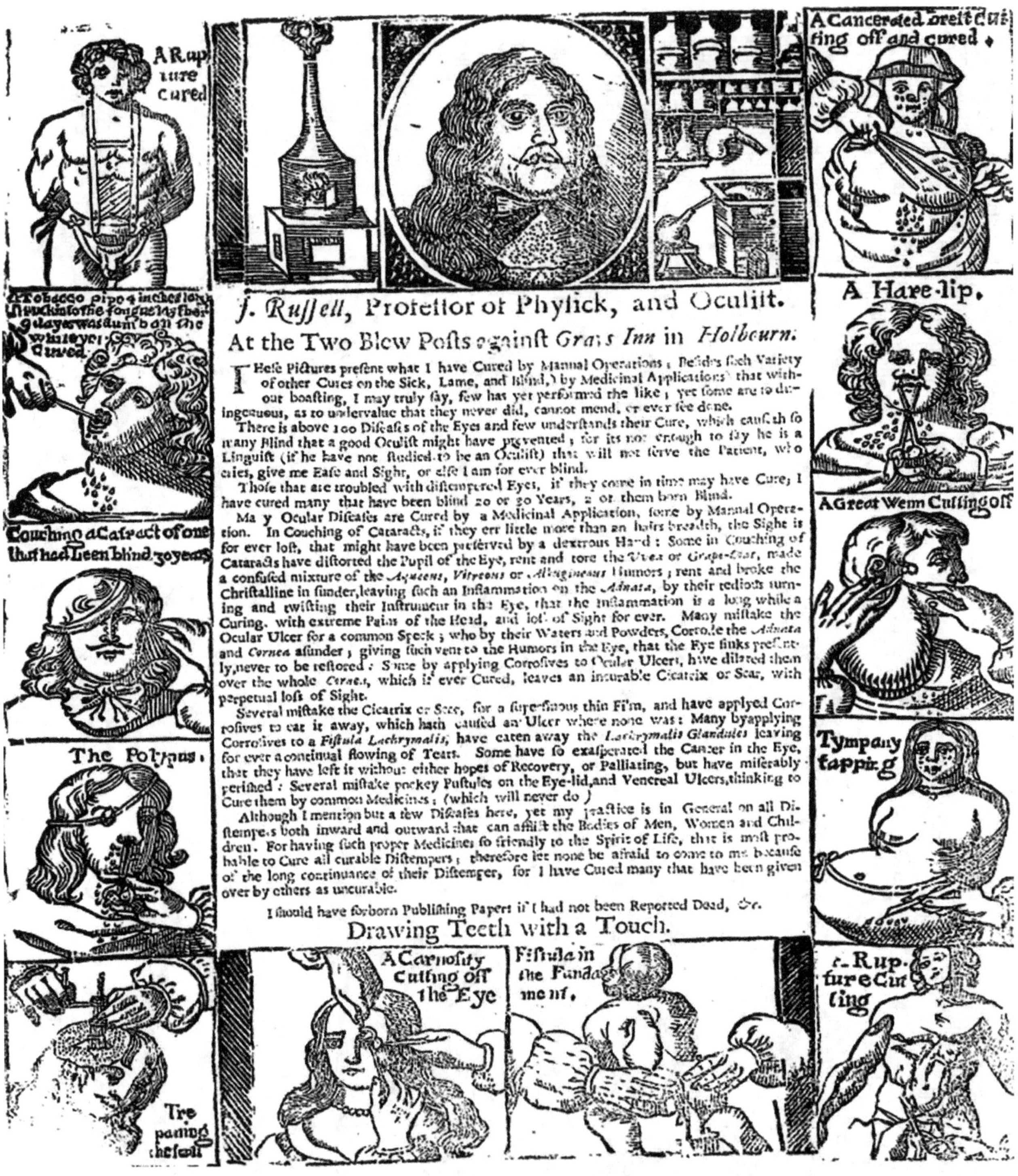

Fig. 14. Surgical procedures performed by John Russell, including cataract couching with the contralateral eye covered, from a handbill dated between 1663 and 1680.

that Russell was licensed by the Archbishop of Canterbury in 1663, the handbill might actually predate Browne's illustration.[198]

Cataract Surgeons and Oculists in Ireland (from 1684)

Early continental medical influences were felt in Ireland. Even though the Romans never captured the island, an oculist stamp from the Roman period found in 1842 at Golden in Tipperary has an inscription interpreted by Freeman to read: "For Marcus Juventus Tutianus a copperas eye salve for old scars."[199] To the best of our knowledge, ancient instruments for cataract couching have not been found in Ireland.

Medieval medical texts from Europe were carried to Ireland, just as they were carried elsewhere in the British Isles. The *Book of the O'Lees*, which dates to about 1434, was written in Gaelic. According to legend, the O'Lees family was given the book by an old man on an enchanted island, which has been suggested to lie in Lough Corrib, Ireland. The description of cataract surgery in this book seems to derive ultimately from Arabic manuscripts. A postoperative plaster with egg yolk (rather than egg white) and oil of viola (or violet oil) is a rather idiosyncratic combination specific to both the *Book of the O'Lees* and Ibn-Sīnā (Avicenna), from about 1020 CE. Of note, in 2018, scholars identified a portion of a 14th-century Gaelic translation of Avicenna stitched to the inside binding of a 16th-century English book. Other couching practices in the *Book of the O'Lees*, such as having the patient sit on a pillow, comforting the patient with kind words during the procedure, and testing the vision during or immediately after the procedure, are not specified in the surviving Greco-Roman texts of Celsus and Paulus Aegineta, but are found in the works of Ibn Īsā (Jesu) and Albucasis.[200] Note that the O'Lees did not specify the patient on a stool or chair, as in many of the later Medieval Latin works. Thus, the legendary old man on the enchanted Irish island probably had at least indirect access to Arabic sources.

Well into the age of the itinerant mountebank, cataract surgery can be documented entering Ireland. The aforementioned visit of English oculist William Read to Trinity College in Dublin in 1684 is the earliest known visit of a cataract surgeon to Ireland. However, apparently by 1687, oculist Richard Reidman had also practiced in Ireland on two occasions.[201] Oculist John Thomas Woolhouse accompanied James II into exile, including a brief period in Ireland, from 1689 to 1690, in which Woolhouse performed paracentesis for hydrophthalmia.[202]

---

198 Leffler et al. "British Isles" 2021.
199 Leffler et al. "British Isles" 2021.
200 Leffler et al. "Annals" 2020.
201 Leffler et al. "British Isles" 2021.
202 Leffler & Schwartz "Woolhouse" 2017.

The earliest identified oculist to live for a prolonged period in Ireland was Mr. Cawood of Dublin, who trained in Paris, and had lived in Ireland beginning about 1700. He was called to Ireland "by a person of Quality, there being none of that profession in that Kingdom."[203] Cawood practiced occasionally in London or Liverpool and was still practicing, apparently in Dublin, in 1722.[204]

Sylvester O'Halloran of Limerick had tried his hand at couching by 1749 and extraction a few times by 1755. He was a general surgeon, licensed at least through 1787.[205]

A great deal of Irish ophthalmic care in the 18th century was handled by itinerants, such as John Taylor, who toured the island several times between 1730 and 1760.[206]

The type of personality that would seek out opportunities at the Western edge of Europe might also be tempted to travel to America. Indeed, William Stork had visited Dublin and Belfast in 1753, before becoming the first cataract coucher in the North American colonies in 1761. Likewise, the 1772 visit to Belfast of Frederick William Jericho of Germany was his last known European stop before traveling to the Caribbean, to become the earliest identified surgeon to perform cataract extraction in the New World by the time of his return in 1776.[207]

The next oculist to settle in Ireland for a prolonged period was Joseph Rouviere (d. 1790), of France. According to Felix Farley's Bristol Journal of June 26, 1762, he was held in the Knowle prison, which held Acadians evacuated from Nova Scotia in 1755. If Rouviere had practiced in Nova Scotia, he would be the earliest cataract surgeon that we know of in French North America. His advertisements merely stated that he had come from Paris and performed cataract extraction in the manner of his teacher, Daviel. He also trained there with Wenzel. Rouviere had moved to Dublin by July 1765, where he had a family and settled down. Rouviere would occasionally tour the island and was still doing cataract surgery in 1787, though he had recently been ill.

Congenital Cataract Surgery: Cheselden's Case (1727)

Congenital cataract surgery played an important role in early British ophthalmology. The procedure was performed as early as 1000 CE by the oculist Ammār ibn 'Alī al-Mawṣilī of Cairo. However, in the Christian world, it was held that congenital blindness could only be healed with a miracle. This belief stemmed from the story

---

203 Leffler et al. "British Isles" 2021.

204 Leffler et al. "British Isles" 2021.

205 Leffler et al. "British Isles" 2021.

206 Leffler et al. "British Isles" 2021.

207 Leffler et al. "British Isles" 2021.

of Jesus curing a man born blind (John 9:32). Ancient Buddhist sutras are also consistent with an understanding of amblyopia.

Nonetheless, such miracles were said to occur in early medieval England. After the miraculous restoration of sight of a peasant's son by Ramelmus, a monk at Much Wenlock in Shropshire in about 1100, the other monks noted that the patient could at first only visually identify those objects that he had previously felt.[208] There is no way to know if the story originated with a cataract surgery, but the description of the outcome raises the possibility.

After clerics were forbidden to perform medical care by the Council of Tours in 1163, such apparent miracles might have been less common. The late 1400s Middle English manuscript of Grassus noted with regard to the incurable *Guttam serenam* with a clear pupil that those "…communly that haue thys Cateracte byth blynde borne."[209]

Patients or doctors might have an incentive to fraudulently claim a miracle had occurred. In 1529, Thomas More (1478-1535) published the story of a beggar from Berwick who claimed to have been miraculously healed of congenital blindness during a visit of King Edward IV (1442-1483) to Saint Albonys. The beggar and his wife insisted that he "cou[l]d neuer se[e] nothi[n]g at all in all hys lyfe before" to Humphrey, the Duke of Gloucester (1390-1447). The beggar was able to name the colors of the Duke's gown and other objects. The Duke pronounced him a fraud, on the basis that the newly sighted might see colors, but would not be able to name them, and had the beggar set in the stocks as punishment. It is hard to see how the tale could be completely accurate, given that the Duke died in 1447, when the king was just 5 years old.[210]

Shakespeare retold the tale in Henry VI, with the Duke of Gloucester saying: "If thou hadst been born blind, thou mightest as well have known all our names as thus to name the several colours we do wear. Sight may distinguish of colours, but suddenly to nominate them all, it is impossible."[211] Shakespeare wrote this play

---

208 Leffler et al. "British Isles" 2021.

209 (Hunter MS 503) Grassus 2011, p. 250. The mid-1400s Hunter MS 513 of Grassus had not mentioned that guttum cerenam was congenital (Grassus 2011, pp. 251-3).

210 Leffler et al. "British Isles" 2021.

211 Henry VI, Part II, Act II, Scene I. James 2013, pp. 226-7. A very similar tale was told in Persia. When Shah Abbas (1571-1629) visited the shrine of the Imam at Meshed, a poor man suddenly claimed to have just had his blindness "from birth" cured by the authority of the saint buried there. The Shah asked the man to name the colors of white and red pieces of cloth, which the man did. The Shah denounced the man as a liar on the basis that it would be impossible to know the names of colors after having vision for only 10 minutes, and the Shah ordered the man's eyes to be plucked out (Elgood C. Safavid Medical Practice. London: Luzac, 1970. p. 67). As no antecedent tale from antiquity or earlier medieval periods is found, the most likely scenario is that the themes in Shakespeare's plays were carried to Safavid Persia.

between 1590 and 1592. At that time, cataract surgery was blossoming in England, but congenital cataract surgery was not known there.

In 1622, Richard Banister compared cataract surgery to Christ's miracles of the Scriptures but believed that "Cataracts in children are uncurable."[212] Banister never claimed to heal congenital blindness.

Shortly after Banister's treatise, secular claims to have healed congenital blindness by cataract surgery appear in England, and in Christendom, for the first time. The earliest congenital cataract surgery that we can find in Western Europe was performed by English oculist John Stepkins, who died in 1652. The surgery, performed in an 18-year-old "Maid" who "lived absolutely blind from the moment of her Birth," was reported by Robert Boyle in 1663. Her postoperative visual function is not specified, but her emotions suggested a positive outcome. She was "ravish at the surprising spectacle of so many and various Objects…that almost everything she saw transported her with admiration and delight."[213] Stepkins learned the oculist trade from his father-in-law, Atwood of Worcester, presumably after marrying his daughter in 1625.[214] Thus, the first congenital cataract surgery in England (and possibly Western Europe) occurred between 1625 and 1652.

Several decades later, surgeons claimed to successfully cure congenital blindness in order to distinguish themselves from their competitors. Oculist John Russell was licensed to practice in 1663, and several of his handbills, which might date from the period 1663 to 1680, advertise cataract couching in those "born blind."[215]

In April 1686, "Doctor Reid and Salvator Moscow, from Sicily," erected stages in Edinburgh and advertised "64 blind persons restored to sight who had never seen from their birth, (which blasphemie out did our Savior's recall miracles, for we read not that he cured so many borne blind)…" This Reid is generally assumed to be the oculist Richard Reidman.[216]

One of the first to regularly advertise congenital cataract surgery was William Read, who also became the earliest identified surgeon to couch cataracts in Ireland in 1684. In 1687, William Read couched the cataract of "the daughter of Mr Johnson at Grundon in Northamptonshire, who was Born Blind and restored to her perfect sight." Read publicized congenital cataract surgeries performed from 1687 onward, including at "Eaton Colledge" in a handbill of 1694. In August 1697, "Dr. William Briggs, Physician in Ordinary to his Majesty" observed Read couch the cataracts

---

212 Banister 1971, np.
213 Leffler et al. "Stepkins" 2014.
214 Leffler & Schwartz "Woolhouse" 2017.
215 Leffler et al. "British Isles" 2021.
216 Leffler et al. "British Isles" 2021.

of a 9-year-old boy named George Smith, who had been born blind. Read continued to perform the procedure through at least 1706.[217]

Others who performed congenital cataract surgery before 1700 included Thomas Clark by 1695, Daubeney Turberville (d. 1696), and Turberville's student Richard Chubb by 1699. In about 1726, Benedict Duddell treated a 7-year-old girl who had been "born blind": "Her Eyes had been needled twice by Dr. Clark...but without success."[218] Duddell was unsuccessful with an additional attempt at couching.

In the late 1600s, congenital cataract surgery began to take on another role—an opportunity to explore the fundamental nature of visual perception. In 1688, William Molyneux (1656-1698) of Ireland proposed in a letter to John Locke that one born blind who suddenly acquired the ability to see would be unable to visually distinguish cubes from spheres, even if these had previously been known by a sense of touch. In 1690, Locke did not directly answer Molyneux's question but did explicitly relate the cure of congenital blindness to cataract surgery:

> "But such an assent upon hearing, no more proves the Ideas to be innate, than it does, That one born blind (with Cataracts, which will be couched to morrow) had the innate Ideas of the Sun, or Light, or Saffron, or Yellow; because when his Sight is cleared, he will certainly assent to this Proposition, That the Sun is lucid [*i.e.* clear], or that Saffron is yellow."[219]

---

217 Leffler et al. "British Isles" 2021.

218 Leffler et al. "British Isles" 2021.

219 Leffler "British Isles" 2021; Locke 1690, "Humane" book I, p. 34. Locke wrote: "Suppose a Child had the use of his Eyes till he knows and distinguishes colours; but then cataracts shut the Windows...This was the case of a blind Man I once talked with, who lost his sight by the small Pox when he was a Child, and had no more notion of colours, than one born Blind...His cataracts are couch'd, and then he has the Ideas...of colours, de novo, by his restor'd sight..." (Locke 1694, "Humane" book I, p. 35) Perhaps, Locke was thinking of John Troughton (c. 1637-1681), who was blinded by smallpox at four years of age, and was at Oxford University from 1655 to 1662 (along with Locke, oxforddnb.com). Troughton went on to become a minister. Locke's writings, such as the 1690 quotation about saffron, could be describing a blind theology scholar. The Bible mentions Saffron only once (Song of Solomon, Ch. 4-6, KJV): "Thy lips are like a thread of scarlet...Spikenard and saffron...fair as the moon, clear as the sun..." In 1678, Troughton paraphrased this passage: "Though the Church be fair as the Moon, she hath also many dark spots; though clear as the Sun, she hath her clouds and Eclipses."(Troughton "Popery" 1680, p. 23) In 1690, Locke recalled: "A studious blind Man... bragg'd one day, That he now understood what Scarlet signified. Upon which his Friend demanding, what Scarlet was? the Blind man answered, It was like the Sound of a Trumpet."(Locke 1690, book III, p. 199) In the "Sermon on Rev. 18.4", Troughton wrote of the papacy: "she [Rome] is arrayed in purple and Scarlet, decked with gold and precious stones and pearls..." (Troughton 1680, "Popery", p. 144). In Revelations 18, we read: "Alas...that great city...clothed in...purple, and scarlet, and decked with gold, and precious stones, and pearls!...And the voice of...trumpeters, shall be heard no more..." (KJV) Revelations 18 is the only Biblical chapter to mention both scarlet and trumpet(er)(s). In 1693, Locke wrote it was "foolish...to set a blind Man to talk of Colours" (Locke "Education" 1693, p. 203). Locke's story should be understood not as synesthesia, but rather as a blind minister struggling to understand Biblical imagery.

In 1694, Locke published Molyneux's question, and wrote that he agreed with Molyneux.

One aspect of Molyneux's biography, which has not been emphasized, is the degree to which he may already have been exposed to oculists who were familiar with congenital cataract surgery. Molyneux married in 1678, and several months later, his wife developed loss of vision. The reputation of oculist Daubeney Turberville of Salisbury extended to Molyneux in Dublin. Therefore, in May 1679, he and his wife traveled to London, where they were evaluated by the oculist Lady Ivy, the daughter of John Stepkins. When she indicated that she could not help them, Molyneux and his wife moved on to Salisbury, where Turberville treated her to no avail. Molyneux and his wife were treated by Turberville a second time in March 1680, this time in London, when Turberville presented the case to royal physician Charles Scarborough, Dr. Richard Lower, and others, who all pronounced the case hopeless. Finally, Molyneux may have crossed paths with Read, who practiced at Trinity College in Dublin in 1684.[220]

In June 1709, oculist Roger Grant was said to have successfully cured a 20-year-old named William Jones, but this case was debunked that year, on the grounds that Jones had a speck on his eye, but was not blind before the treatment, and could not see much better afterward. Moreover, a certificate from the Minister verifying the oculist's claims was forged.[221]

In 1709, Irish cleric and philosopher George Berkeley (1685-1753) agreed with Molyneux that one suddenly brought to sight would not be able to visually distinguish cubes from spheres and added that the patient would also not be able to immediately judge distance and magnitude.[222]

Conventional accounts stipulate that the first credible, empirical evidence regarding Molyneux's question came from the 1728 report of English surgeon William Cheselden, who was said to have restored to sight a boy who was born blind. This case has been discussed by prominent philosophers such as Diderot and Buffon over the past three centuries. In 1738, Voltaire (1694-1778) wrote that Cheselden's patient was reluctant to consent, but that "the operation was however performed, and fully succeeded. The youth, then about fourteen years of age, saw the light for the first time. This experiment confirmed all that Locke and Barclay [Berkeley] had justly foreseen."[223] Cheselden's remains one of the most highly cited case reports from centuries ago. However, we have obtained new information that might call this case into question.

---

220 Leffler et al. "British Isles" 2021.
221 James 2013, pp. 230-1.
222 Leffler et al. "British Isles" 2021.
223 Leffler et al. "British Isles" 2021.

None of these discussants has known the family story or the name of Cheselden's patient, whom we have now identified. The patient's father, Daniel Dolins, Esq, studied philosophy and mathematics with Johannes Luyts of Utrecht in 1697. The senior Dolins returned to London and, in 1700, married Margaret, the daughter of Thomas Cooke of Hackney (d. 1694). Dolins was knighted in 1722.[224]

Dolins and his wife Margaret had four children: Abraham (b. 1701), Mary (b. 1703/4), Daniel (b. 1713), and Margaret (b. 1715). Both sons had bilateral cataracts and died as young adults. Daniel, the son, was Cheselden's patient.

Abraham was operated for one of his congenital cataracts at age 13. By 1721, surgery for congenital cataracts had been performed on children as early as age 18 months in Paris by Woolhouse (Figs. 15 and 16). However, it was more common to defer surgery until affected children were older. In a letter of October 11, 1714, the father informed clergyman John Strype (1643-1737):

> It pleased God to afflict our Eldest Son with Cataracts in both Eyes from his Birth. We design God willing to have him Couched in one of them by Mrs. Jones on Thursday next.[225]

Mrs. Jones was from a family that had been practicing as oculists since the mid-1600s. On October 15, 1714, Dolins updated Strype:

> ...the operation was yesterday very well perform'd by the Divine Assistance, & the Child is as well as we can expect in so short a time, but we must wait with some Patience for the ripening & dissolving of the matter before he can have his clean sight ...[226]

Pediatric cataracts are typically soft and would probably break up during an attempted couching before being gradually absorbed. In May 1715, Dolins informed Strype:

> Mrs. Jones designs God Willing on Wednesday next to renew the operation on one of my sons eyes in order to remove some remaining strings which obstruct his Perfect Sight...These are therefore to desire you to renew your Prayers...[to] make this second operation completely successful.[227]

Mrs. Jones died in 1720, but her legacy was carried on by a succession of women oculists who passed on her knowledge.[228]

---

224 Leffler et al. "British Isles" 2021.

225 Leffler et al. "British Isles" 2021.

226 Leffler et al. "British Isles" 2021.

227 Leffler et al. "British Isles" 2021.

228 Leffler et al. "British Isles" 2021.

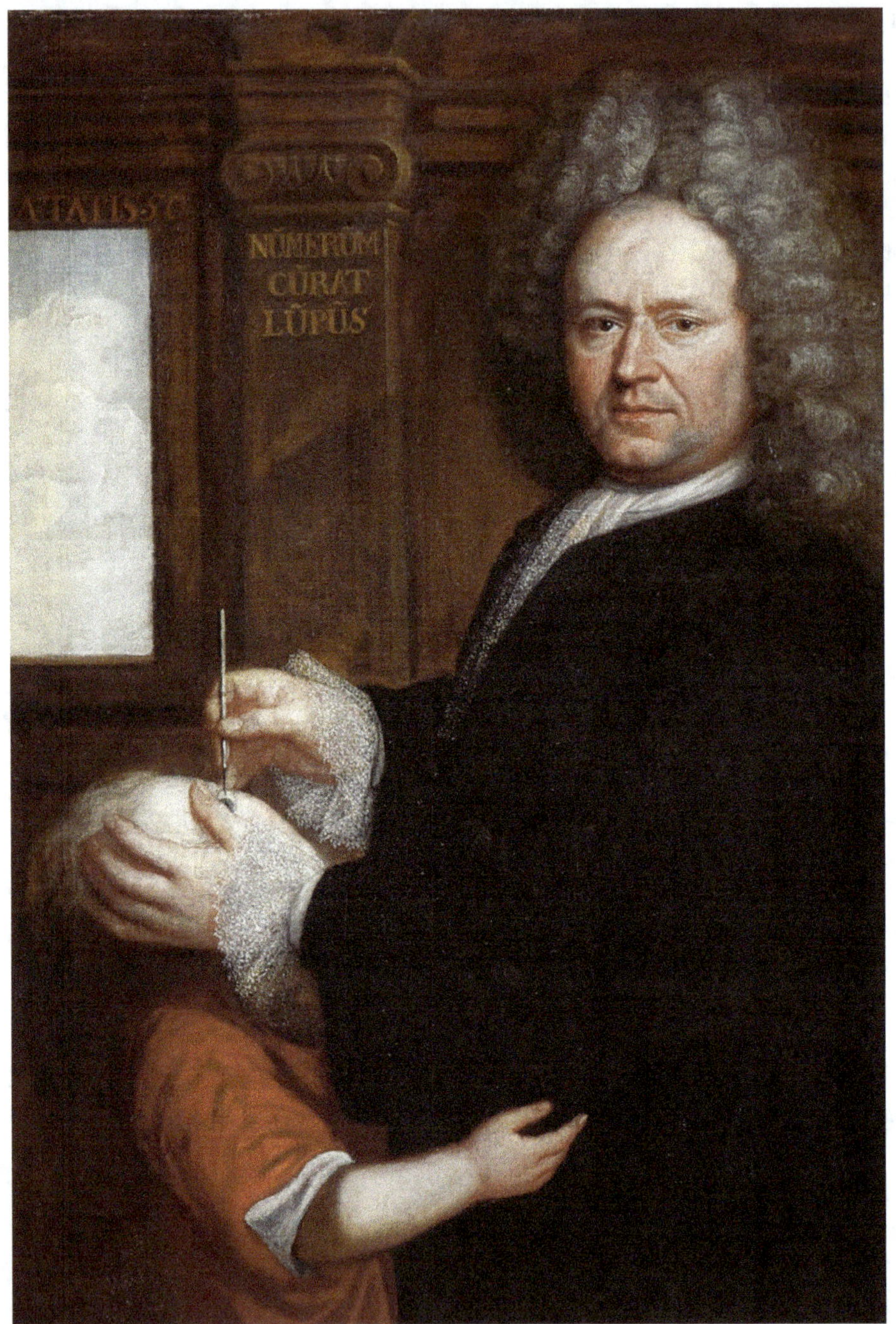

Fig. 15. An anonymous painting "Portret van de oogarts François De Wulf," from Bruges, dated to 1700, showing cataract couching in a child.

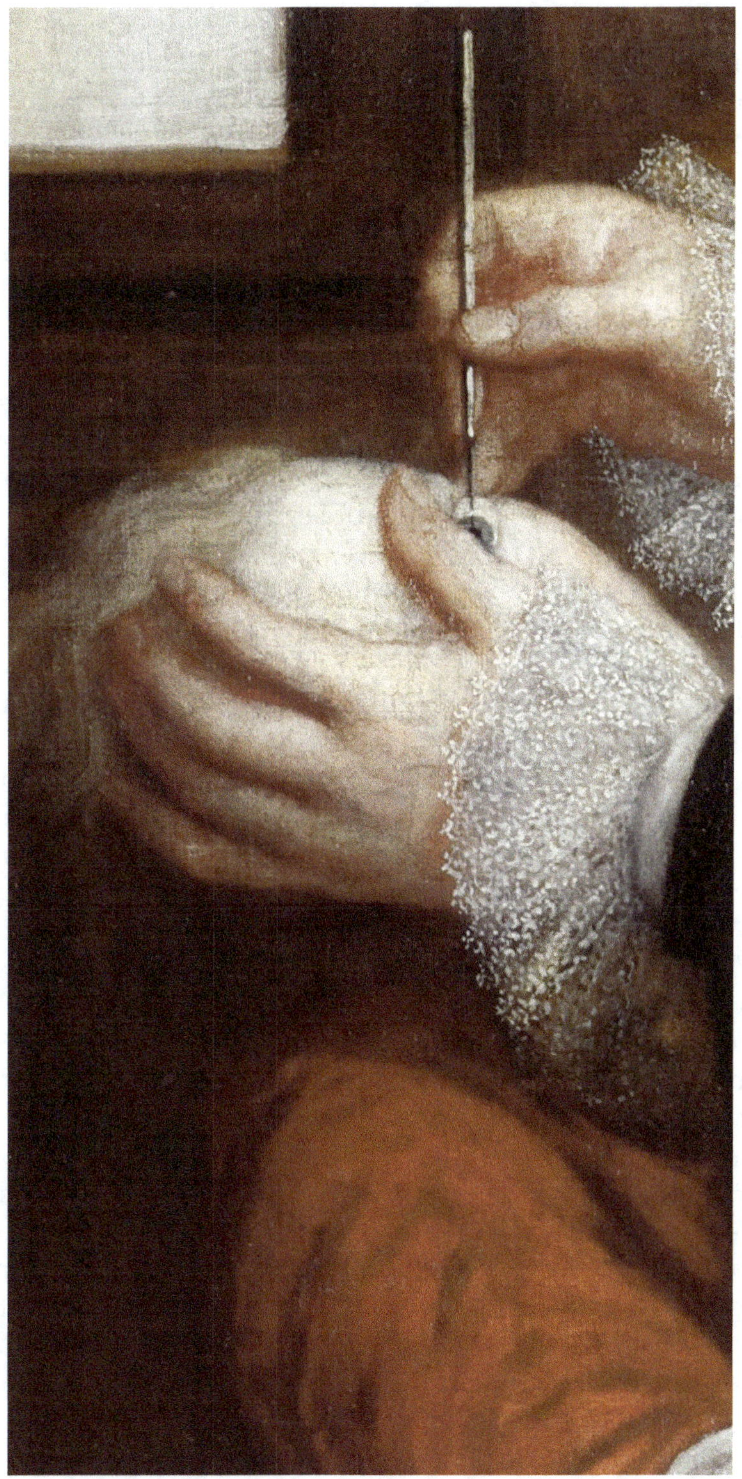

Fig. 16. Detail of the portrait of cataract surgery by François De Wulf dated to 1700 showing that the needle appears to pass close to the pars plana, but anterior to the iris.

Congenital cataracts are sometimes associated with developmental disability, but there is no evidence of intellectual disability in the Dolins children. When Mary died at age 16 in February 1719/1720, the family minister, Daniel Mayo, recalled that she "was desirous to instruct her younger Brother and Sister…And delighted to converse about religious Matters with her Brother [Abraham], that was older than herself."[229] Mary had suffered for some time from "Consumption," with pain and "frequent Coughing." Her eyes were apparently fine, as even to the end, she read the Bible and Mr. Baxter's *Dying Thoughts*.[230] Her brother Abraham also died in 1720, when he was 19 years old.

Dolins, Berkeley, and Cheselden belonged to the same social networks. The fact that Berkeley was directly linked with the family of Cheselden's patient (the Dolins family) was not recognized before our research. Moreover, the social ties between Berkeley and Cheselden had not been explored.

The senior Dolins was one of the Governours of St. Thomas's Hospital from 1714 to 1725. Surgeon William Cheselden joined the hospital staff in 1718.[231]

Berkeley spent most of the years 1724 through 1728 in London and was elected to the Society for Promotion of Christian Knowledge (SPCK) in 1725. The senior Dolins had been a member of this Society since 1710 and appears to have made Berkeley's acquaintance. Berkeley planned to found a university in Bermuda, which he would lead as president. Berkeley established a committee of prominent citizens who could receive contributions for this effort. Berkeley's committee, announced on July 15, 1725, included "Sir Daniel Dolins, Kt." He also included the "Rev. Dr. [Richard] Mayo, Treasurer to the S.P.C.K., at St. Thomas's Hospital," the brother of the Dolins family minister.[232] Berkeley's committee also included "John Arbuthnot, MD," a friend of Cheselden with whom Berkeley had previously corresponded and also discussed philosophy while visiting Arbuthnot's lodging for dinner.[233]

The poet Alexander Pope was one of the closest friends of both Berkeley and Cheselden. In 1722, Pope requested that Cheselden write down lines from Shakespeare that Cheselden had mentioned to Arbuthnot. In fact, Cheselden played a role in editing Pope's 1725 edition of Shakespeare. While preparing the book, Pope wrote to a colleague: "Let friend Cheselden be of ye party." Even though Cheselden was his doctor, Pope referred to him as "friend Cheselden" several times. Pope frequently ate dinner at Cheselden's home, and when Pope needed medical treatment in 1736, Pope stayed there. Pope implied that Cheselden advised him about his own

---

229 Leffler et al. "British Isles" 2021.

230 Leffler et al. "British Isles" 2021.

231 Leffler et al. "British Isles" 2021.

232 Leffler et al. "British Isles" 2021.

233 Leffler et al. "British Isles" 2021.

eyes and notified Cheselden when there were cataracts to be operated on in Bath. Cheselden was with Pope during his final illness.[234]

Berkeley was also very close with Pope. The two met in 1713 when both contributed essays to Steele's *Guardian*. One of Pope's *Guardian* essays mirrors the themes in Berkeley's *New Theory of Vision*, suggesting that Pope had read it, even though it had only been published in Dublin. Berkeley and Pope shared dinner with a friend in 1721, when Berkeley stayed with Pope for a week. Pope invited Berkeley, writing: "As I take You to be almost the only Friend I have, that is above the little vanities of the Town…" During 1726 and 1727 when Berkeley was putting together funding for his proposed Bermuda college, he asked Pope to translate a poem, some lines from which Berkeley inserted in his Bermuda literature.[235]

One joint acquaintance of Berkeley and Cheselden who ultimately publicized the surgery was Voltaire, who, while living in London from 1726 to 1728, also met with Pope and the Princess of Wales. Voltaire later wrote that he "had seen a great deal of Cheselden," and handwrote a dedication to Cheselden in his 1738 *Philosophie*. Voltaire also wrote that "…the celebrated Cheselden, one of the greatest surgeons in London, told me that it was he who first caused them [surgical instruments] to be manufactured in that city, in 1715." Likewise, Voltaire indicated that he discussed philosophy several times with Berkeley while in England.[236]

Berkeley had originally met Caroline, the Princess of Wales (1683-1737), in 1712, after his earliest philosophical works were published. It is conceivable that the philosophical implications of Molyneux's question would have come up early in their relationship, given that Berkeley had just published on the question and that they were introduced by Molyneux's son Samuel. During this London period, from 1724 to 1728, Berkeley debated philosophy and theology weekly in front of the intellectual Caroline.[237]

Perhaps, it was between 1722 and 1725 when Cheselden became interested in eye surgery. Cheselden's 1722 edition of his anatomy text mentioned cataract couching in passing, whereas the earlier edition did not. Students who finished their training with him before 1722 did not become known for eye surgery or teaching, while subsequent trainees did. During this period, cataract surgery was still largely in the hands of dedicated oculists, and the volume of general surgeons such as Cheselden was typically quite low. The yearlong logbook of a student named Charles Oxley who was training at St. Thomas's Hospital records several cataract surgeries at the hospital, beginning in May 1725. In one case, performed successfully in a 30-year-old man in June 1725, Oxley recorded that Cheselden was the surgeon.

---

234 Leffler et al. "British Isles" 2021.

235 Leffler et al. "British Isles" 2021.

236 Leffler et al. "British Isles" 2021.

237 Leffler et al. "British Isles" 2021.

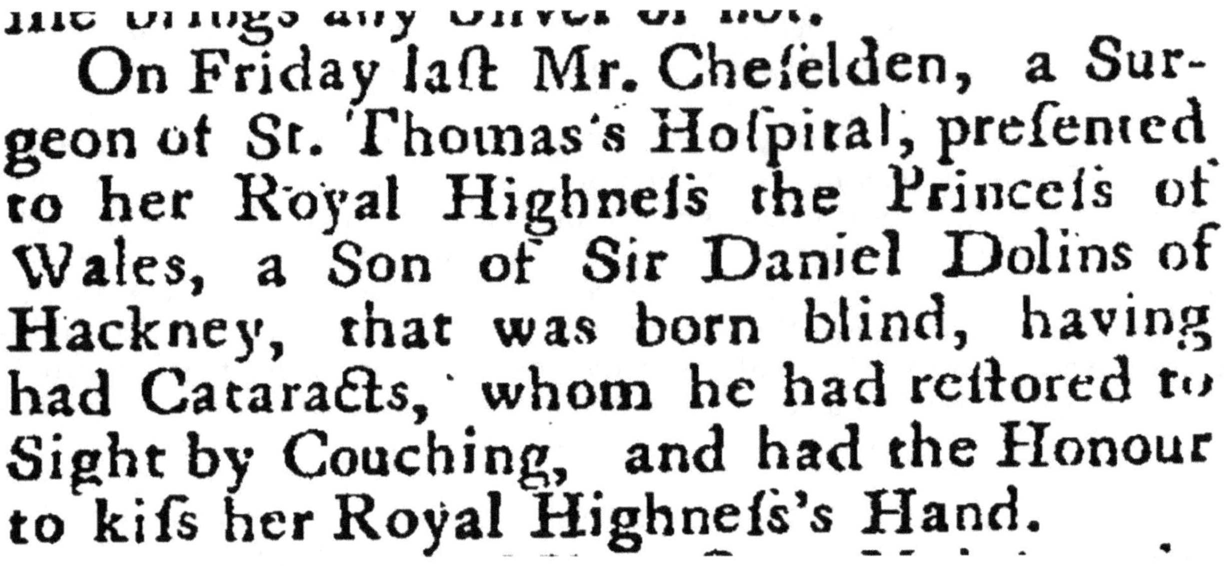

On Friday laſt Mr. Cheſelden, a Surgeon of St. Thomas's Hoſpital, preſented to her Royal Highneſs the Princeſs of Wales, a Son of Sir Daniel Dolins of Hackney, that was born blind, having had Cataraɛts, whom he had reſtored to Sight by Couching, and had the Honour to kiſs her Royal Highneſs's Hand.

Fig. 17. Illustration showing Mr. Cheselden has performed a cataract couching in Daniel Dolins (the son) who "was born blind," in the *Daily Journal* of March 14, 1727.

Daniel Dolins (the son) was born on April 2, 1713. On March 14, 1727, the *Daily Journal* contained the first public notice of any eye surgery by Cheselden:

> ...Mr. Cheselden, a Surgeon of St. Thomas's Hospital, presented to her Royal Highness the Princess of Wales, a Son of Sir Daniel Dolins of Hackney, that was born blind, having had Cataracts, whom he had restored to Sight by Couching, and had the Honour to kiss her Royal Highness's Hand.[238]

Historians have not previously noticed this newspaper report that permits us to identify Daniel Dolins as Cheselden's famous patient (Fig. 17). In October 1727, Caroline was crowned queen following the death of King George I. In December 1727, Cheselden was named the surgeon to Queen Caroline.[239]

Cheselden's only ophthalmic publications (outside the chapter on the eye in his anatomy treatise) were two curious reports published together in 1728 in the *Philosophical Transactions of the Royal Society of London*.[240] The first report concerned the perceptions and emotions of a 13-year-old boy, who had been blind from a young age and was then couched. The patient was referred to as a "gentleman," as one would expect for the son of a knight.

---

238 No author listed, Daily Journal, March 14, 1727, p. 1.

239 Leffler et al. "British Isles" 2021.

240 Cheselden 1728; Leffler et al. "British Isles" 2021.

In the 1730 edition of his anatomy text, Cheselden included this report and wrote:

> I have couched several others who were born blind, whose observations were of the same kind; but they being younger, none of them gave so full an account as this gentleman.[241]

This note helps to establish that the 1728 report was about Daniel, because the small number of other children operated on by Cheselden were younger.

An analysis of this 1728 report reveals that (1) although the tone of the report implies that Daniel could see better, it is not actually specified that he could perform additional visual tasks, and (2) the report used language more characteristic of Berkeley than of Cheselden. To illustrate the latter, we have italicized words used in Berkeley's writings, but never used by Cheselden (in a database of period texts).[242]

The report was ambiguous about whether Daniel's visual dysfunction was congenital. The report described "a *young Gentleman*, who was born blind, or lost his Sight so early, that he had no *Remembrance* of ever having seen." Both the newspaper notice mentioning Cheselden and Cheselden's anatomy text addendum implied that Daniel was "born blind." He was blind from his "infancy" according to Berkeley. Daniel was blind from the age of about 2 years, according to the most unbiased source—his longtime tutor.[242]

The author suggested that Daniel could see better postoperatively by including vague statements, such as alluding to the postoperative period "when he first saw…" In addition, "A Year after first Seeing," Daniel said he had "a *new Kind* of Seeing."[243]

Daniel anticipated he would someday be able to perform numerous visual tasks: reading, writing, walking *"abroad."* The reader might suppose that eventually Daniel could perform some of these tasks. In fact, no improvement in performance of any visual task is specified. The report was clear that even several months after the surgery, Daniel could not visually distinguish a cat from a dog. We know from Daniel's tutor that Daniel was never able to read.[244]

Peter Kennedy, a surgeon who had spoken with "the parent" of Daniel, wrote in 1739: "…far from being able to read or write therewith…It seems even to be with considerable difficulty he can guide himself along without some Assistance; and… he still knows Puss…much better by his feeling than he does by his seeing."[245]

---

241 Leffler et al. "British Isles" 2021.

242 Leffler et al. "British Isles" 2021.

243 Leffler et al. "British Isles" 2021.

244 Leffler et al. "British Isles" 2021.

245 Leffler et al. "British Isles" 2021.

Daniel's positive emotions after surgery were mentioned in the 1728 report, apparently in an attempt to suggest improved vision. Referring to Cheselden in the third person, the author related Daniel's emotions:

> ...his *Gratitude* to his Operator he could not *conceal*, never seeing him for some Time without Tears of *Joy* in his Eyes, and other Marks of *Affection*: And if he did not happen to come at any Time when he was expected, he would be so *griev'd*, that he *could not forbear* crying at his Disappointment.[246]

How could Cheselden know what occurred in his absence?

The 1728 report was signed "Chesselden," which varied from how he spelled his name in his publications.[247] The fact that the 1728 report was narrated in the plural form ("we") suggests that it might have been a multi-author work. Elsewhere, we have demonstrated that the report used Berkeley's language (and not Cheselden's) regarding emotions, mental, or sensory processes and other idiosyncratic expressions.[248]

The observations of the 13-year-old Daniel were suspiciously similar to those of Berkeley. It was not until "about 2 months" after surgery that Daniel discovered that pictures "represented solid Bodies," instead of "Party-colour'd Planes, or Surfaces diversified with Variety of Paint." In 1709, Berkeley had written: "What we strictly see are not Solids, nor yet Plains variously colour'd; they are only Diversity of Colours."[249] Daniel "ask'd which was the lying Sense, Feeling, or Seeing?" Berkeley frequently reviewed the teachings of the philosopher Heraclitus, who "used to call...eyesight a lying sense."[250]

The 13-year-old Daniel thought objects looked "extremely large." Daniel's interlocutor found him:

> never being able to imagine any Lines *beyond* the *Bounds* he saw; the Room he was in he said, he knew to be but Part of the House, yet he could not conceive that the whole House could look bigger.[251]

Who asked Daniel at his home whether he could imagine lines extending beyond the bounds he saw? Here is Berkeley writing about mathematics:

> ...the Mind finds no difficulty in conceiving them [mathematical expressions] to be continued *beyond* any assignable *Bounds*.[252]

---

246 Leffler et al. "British Isles" 2021.
247 Cheselden 1728.
248 Leffler et al. "British Isles" 2021.
249 Leffler et al. "British Isles" 2021.
250 Leffler et al. "British Isles" 2021.
251 Cheselden 1728.
252 Leffler et al. "British Isles" 2021.

Elsewhere, Berkeley wrote:

> Mathematicians...do not conceive or imagine Lines or Surfaces less than what are perceivable to the Sense.[253]

Daniel's preoperative perception of colors is described in the 1728 report as only producing *faint Ideas* in his mind. Berkeley, who viewed real objects as only existing in the mind, repeatedly described ideas as being faint. In 1733, Berkeley claimed that his theories about perceptions after sudden acquisition of vision were "not a little confirmed" by the 1728 report.[254]

We actually learn more about the clinical course from Kennedy, who wrote that "six months after the operation on the last eye," the child "felt something in his Eye, which seemed to him to give a Crack." The globe was inflamed and painful, with turbid aqueous humor, and "a great Flux of a watery Humour, probably from the Lachrymal Gland."[255] Kennedy supposed that the clinical picture might have been due to rupture of the crystalline lens. Perhaps, the cornea perforated.

The accompanying report by Cheselden in the 1728 Transactions concerned the production of "an Incision thro' the Iris" (iridotomy) in two eyes. This report is written in a completely different style, and there is no reason to doubt Cheselden's authorship. Cheselden matter-of-factly recounts how he cut the iris in the first person singular ("I"), without mentioning the patients' emotions.[256]

In 1728, Sir Daniel Dolins passed away. Also, George Berkeley got married and headed for America, intending to start his Bermuda college. The 1728 report ultimately became influential when Voltaire publicized it in France, and the report of "Chesselden" continues to be cited liberally in the modern era.[257]

However, the funds for Berkeley's Bermuda college were never disbursed by the government, and Berkeley returned to London in 1731. In 1734, he wrote that he no longer attended (Caroline's) court. It was surgeon John Ranby, rather than Cheselden, who was asked to attend to Queen Caroline when she was dying from a hernia.[258]

The 1728 report on recovery from congenital blindness must have interested John Eames (1686-1744), a fellow of the Royal Society. Eames was a clergyman who taught the writings of John Locke, as well as anatomy as early as 1617, and helped to lead the Fund Academy that trained dissenting clergymen. This academy

---

253 Leffler et al. "British Isles" 2021.

254 Leffler et al. "British Isles" 2021.

255 Leffler et al. "British Isles" 2021.

256 Leffler et al. "British Isles" 2021.

257 Leffler et al. "British Isles" 2021.

258 Leffler et al. "British Isles" 2021.

subsequently placed tutors in Daniel's home for the remainder of his life. We can assume that Daniel's continued poor vision was familiar to Eames by 1734, when he edited an abridged version of the Transactions, which included the 1728 report about Daniel.[259]

Daniel's first tutor was William Ford, who left to become ordained as a minister in December 1730. Eames replaced Ford with Isaac Toms (1710-1801), who lived with the family for 11 years. Toms' memoirs recounted: "From the age of two years, this amiable youth [Daniel] had been almost blind; a circumstance which greatly increased the labour of Mr. Toms, who constantly read to, or conversed with him, eight hours in the day, on the subjects of religion or science."[260] Toms did not mention Daniel's eye surgeries, perhaps because they had no significant impact on his vision. It is unlikely that this omission resulted from a lack of interest on the part of Toms, who when young had studied anatomy and considered becoming a surgeon.

Toms was still living with the family in September 1742 when a friend wrote, sending his regards to Mr. Dolins, and recounting how the oculist John Taylor, a former Cheselden student, was healing the blind in Bath.[261]

The cataracts in the Dolins brothers were probably hereditary, but it is unlikely that the precise cause can be determined after three centuries. The absence of reports of vision impairment in prior generations is consistent with autosomal recessive inheritance. The premature deaths of the Dolins brothers might have been unrelated to the cataracts. Multiple genes, including variants in the crystalline genes, are associated with nonsyndromic (isolated), inherited congenital cataracts. Some of these variants can be manifest in an autosomal recessive manner.[262]

Still, it is tempting to speculate on a single disorder to explain the brothers' entire clinical picture. Sengers syndrome is an autosomal recessive disorder, resulting in cataracts that are typically congenital (as in Abraham's case) but can occur at a few years of age (as may have occurred in Daniel's case). Sengers syndrome is associated with normal mental development, hypertrophic cardiomyopathy, skeletal myopathy, and lactic acidosis. The syndrome can result in chronic disability, followed, in its milder form, by death near the third decade of life, as occurred in the Dolins brothers. The initial series, and many subsequent cases, have been reported from the Netherlands, whence Sir Daniel Dolins' family hailed. In Iceland, the prevalence is about 1 in 40,000.[263]

Kennedy, who knew Cheselden personally, thought the emphasis on visual physiology in the 1730 edition of Cheselden's anatomy text, which reprinted the 1728

---

259 Leffler et al. "British Isles" 2021.
260 Leffler et al. "British Isles" 2021.
261 Leffler et al. "British Isles" 2021.
262 Leffler et al. "British Isles" 2021.
263 Leffler et al. "British Isles" 2021.

report about Daniel, was out of character for the surgically minded Cheselden. Kennedy accused Cheselden of writing it "with the Advice and Assistance of his Friends."[264] Berkeley is known to have published other writings anonymously or with a pseudonym.[265]

We may never know with certainty whether Berkeley wrote the report describing the eye surgery in his colleague's son. But the report is certainly misleading. Whereas the report suggests that the cataracts might have been congenital, the most unbiased source (Daniel's tutor) states the vision loss began at about 2 years of age. Most importantly, there is no evidence that the surgery helped Daniel to read or perform visual tasks. Therefore, the report cannot provide evidence regarding the perceptions of one suddenly acquiring vision, despite its centrality to the philosophical debates over the past three centuries. Congenital cataract surgery is a flawed model to answer the Molyneux question, because congenital cataract patients often have some (albeit reduced) visual function to begin with, and because dense amblyopia precludes the sudden acquisition of perfect vision with surgery. Berkeley was probably correct that one suddenly gaining vision would have difficulty visually distinguishing objects familiar from a sense of touch, though there is still some debate.[266] However, Berkeley's claim that his theories were proved by the report is inconsistent with the clinical reality that Daniel truly lived.

Daniel Dolins had wanted to purchase a country estate to erect a chapel. However, his plans did not come to fruition, and he died in July 1743:

> On Tuesday last died Daniel Dolins, Esq...A Gentleman as generally esteem'd as known; who, with all that was obliging had good Sense and Furniture of Mind...He was an ardent Lover of Truth, and under peculiar Disadvantages, arising from a Defect of Sight, search'd diligently for it...He died after a long illness...but not till he had said, a little before Death, My Sufferings are nothing, and I am happy.[267]

Traditional Surgeons at Hospitals (1720s-1800)

As noted earlier, families and mountebanks were the major sources of ophthalmic instruction in the British Isles during the 17th century. Despite the initial early efforts to couch cataracts by traditional surgeons in Oxford and Glasgow, there is little evidence that the practice became sustained among this group during the 17th century. We do not find evidence of cataract surgery taught at hospitals staffed by traditional surgeons until the 18th century.

---

264 Leffler et al. "British Isles" 2021.

265 Leffler et al. "British Isles" 2021.

266 Leffler et al. "British Isles" 2021.

267 Leffler et al. "British Isles" 2021.

It is true that when surgeon Alexander Read (1586-1641) lectured at "Chirurgeans Hall" in London from 1632 to 1634, he reviewed cataract couching and, in 1638, mentioned that the aqueous humor would return after paracentesis in men, or in chickens, over the course of 15 days.[268]

Joseph Binns (d. 1664) performed his apprenticeship with Joseph Fenton and was a surgeon at St. Bartholomew's Hospital from 1647 until his death. Binns' casebooks describe 671 patients and do not mention cataract couching, though he did treat three corneal ulcers, one with blistering, purging, cupping, and medicines dropped in the eye.[269] Likewise, the observations of James Molins, a student at St. Thomas's Hospital from 1674 to 1677, do not mention cataract couching.

William Briggs was sometimes called an oculist due to his interest in medical treatments of the eyes. Still, the mainstream physicians viewed the itinerants as the experts in eye surgery. As noted earlier, Briggs observed Read perform a congenital cataract surgery in 1697.

In the 1720s and 1730s, evidence emerges of cataract couching in hospitals: William Cheselden at St. Thomas's Hospital, Samuel Palmer and John Freke at St. Bartholomew's Hospital, John Ranby at St. George's Hospital, Samuel Sharp at Guy's Hospital, and Cheselden and Thomas Hope at the Westminster Infirmary.[270]

Even if many of the hospital-based or hospital-trained general surgeons did not have the surgical volume or skill of the specialist itinerant oculists, the entry of eye surgery into the hospitals did have important influences on the overall development of ophthalmology. Cataract couching became the domain of a significant fraction of general surgeons. The surgeries were performed indoors, rather than on an outdoor stage. The general surgeons were typically attached to a given hospital and would be available to manage postoperative complications, even months or years later. An apprentice bound to one surgeon was free to observe surgeries performed by other attendings at the hospital. In fact, apprentices at St. Thomas's Hospital or Guy's Hospital could attend surgeries at either hospital. Moreover, one attending might assist a fellow attending surgeon. Although some of the larger itinerant productions also had served as educational institutions of a sort, they were unlikely to outlast the dominant personality. In contrast, the hospitals had institutional memory, which would outlast any given surgeon, and thereby provided continuity.

Some prominent patients were couched by traditional surgeons in this era. In 1752, Samuel Sharp of Guy's Hospital attempted to couch the cataract of the

---

268 Leffler et al. "British Isles" 2021.
269 Leffler et al. "British Isles" 2021.
270 Leffler et al. "British Isles" 2021.

46-year-old poet Anna Williams (1706-1783) but found that it was too soft. On November 3, 1752, composer "George-Frederick Handel, Esq; was couch'd by William Bromfield, Esq; Surgeon to her Royal Highness the Princess of Wales."[271]

Still, the traditional surgeons continued to look to itinerant oculists as teachers. Surgeon Richard Kay (1716-1751) observed John Taylor perform eye surgeries on a visit to Manchester in July 1742 before training at Guy's Hospital.[272] William Hey of Leeds had trained with London surgeons, but he never performed cataract surgery himself until 1768, the same year, Hilmer visited his city and demonstrated a small round couching needle to him. Similarly, surgeon James Lucas of Leeds observed Hilmer perform couching in 1769.[273]

Cataract Extraction (by 1753)

It was in the latter half of the 18th century that planned cataract extraction was performed by some surgeons. Before cataract extraction could be routinely practiced, surgeons had to figure out that a cataract was an opacity of the crystalline lens. Since antiquity, it had been believed that the cataract was an opacity anterior to the lens. The correct understanding became widely known in the first half of the 18th century in Paris. Some British students, such as Benedict Duddell, traveled to Paris to study with John Thomas Woolhouse, who did admit after 1715 that the structure being couched was an opaque crystalline lens, though he insisted on calling the diseased lens a "glaucoma."[274]

In about 1713, Mr. Cawood couched a Dubliner with partial success, and when the patient died in 1722, Thomas Molyneux dissected the eye and found neither a membrane nor the crystalline lens and surmised that the lens had been absorbed.[275]

Surgical student Charles Oxley recorded in May 1725 that William Cheselden at St. Thomas's Hospital had dissected a cadaver with a cataract to confirm that the entire crystalline lens was opaque. In his treatise of 1727, John Taylor claimed to have discovered that the cataract was an opacity of the lens but credited Cheselden with laying the groundwork for this discovery.[276]

---

271 Leffler et al. "British Isles" 2021.

272 As an aside, Kay assaulted a fellow student in Guy's Hospital who accused him of sexual impropriety. Shortly thereafter, Kay's professors determined that he was ready to graduate and go back to his hometown! Kay only performed one unsuccessful couching and died young (Leffler et al. "British Isles" 2021).

273 Leffler et al. "British Isles" 2021.

274 Leffler et al. "British Isles" 2021.

275 Leffler et al. "British Isles" 2021.

276 Leffler et al. "British Isles" 2021.

In the early 1700s, when the lens happened to sublux into the anterior chamber during couching, it would be removed by surgeons, such as John Thomas Woolhouse in Paris and John Taylor of England. It can be documented that Jacques Daviel of France performed planned cataract extraction by 1750.[277] Daviel made a small inferior corneal limbal incision, which was then extended using right and left curved scissors. He also disrupted the lens capsule, to extract the lens without its capsule (extracapsular extraction).

After Daviel's presentation of planned cataract extraction, Samuel Sharp was an early adopter. However, Sharp made several modifications in one patient on April 7, 1753, and presented his experience to the Royal Society of London 5 days later. First, he made the inferior corneal incision with a single knife. Second, Sharp advocated removing the lens intact in its capsule (intracapsular extraction), with the lens expelled by pressure. If pressure did not suffice, Sharp impaled the lens with his knife to remove the lens still in its capsule. Although his surgical textbook became quite popular, it is not clear that any high-volume surgeons or oculists had success with the intracapsular technique. In fact, after 1758, Sharp preferred couching, and suspended judgment on cataract extraction until more was known. The closest we see to an oculist adopting intracapsular extraction might be Frederick Bischoff, who noted that one could apply gentle pressure, but if this failed, a capsulorhexis was performed.[278]

In fact, few generalist surgeons trained in the British Isles had success with cataract extraction. Thomas Young (d. 1783) of the Royal Infirmary at Edinburgh published six cataract extractions using an extracapsular technique, initially with apparent success. However, within a few months, the sight was lost, and Young soured on extraction in general. Joseph Warner (1717-1801) of London was familiar with both couching and extraction by 1754, but in 1760, he wrote: "…I am inclined to believe that the Operation of Couching will still prevail." By the end of the century, only about half the cataract surgeons in the British Isles were known to perform cataract extraction (Fig. 18). This is slightly higher than the one-third known to perform cataract extraction in the United States.[279]

As in the heyday of couching, the English surgeons looked to foreign itinerant oculists as authorities regarding cataract surgery. In 1785, Benjamin Bell of Edinburgh favored couching, and though he was familiar with patients who had had cataract extraction, it was not totally clear that he had personally performed the procedure. However, in 1787, the ophthalmic sections of his treatise had been heavily edited to reflect what he had learned from assisting Jean François Pellier in cataract extractions.[280]

---

277 Leffler et al. "Daviel" 2023.

278 Leffler et al. "British Isles" 2021.

279 Leffler et al. "British Isles" 2021.

280 Leffler et al. "British Isles" 2021.

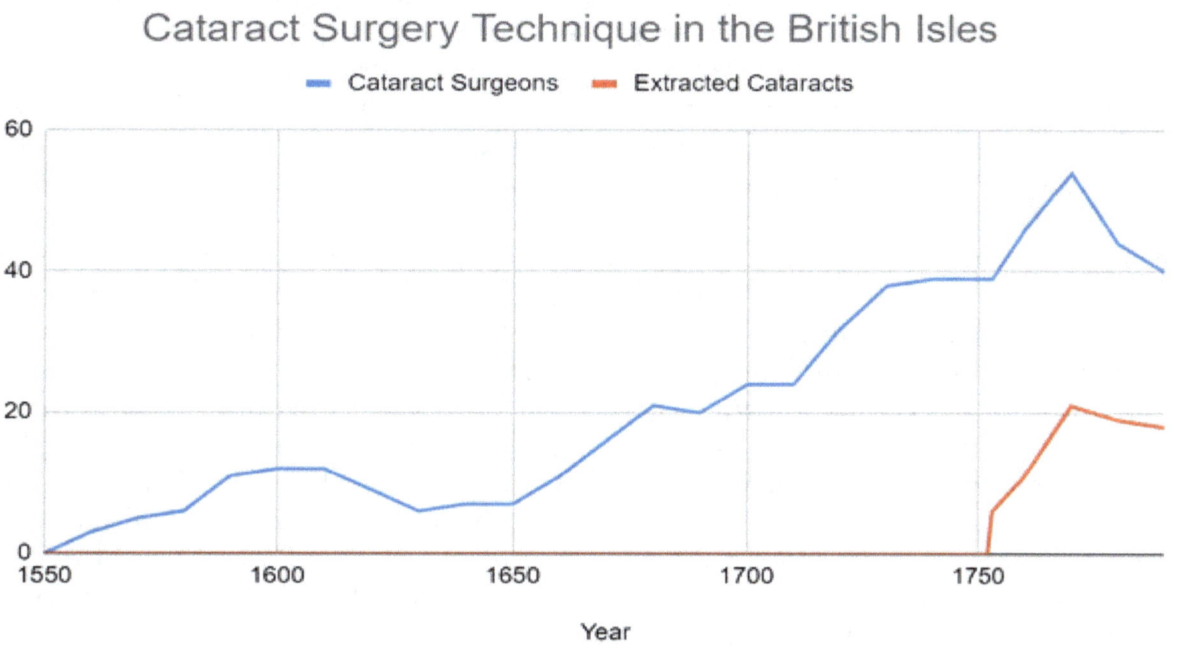

Fig. 18. Number of total cataract surgeons in the British Isles (blue line) and number of surgeons performing cataract extraction (red line) during each decade.

In 1768, Sharp and Thomas Gataker observed Baron Wenzel perform bilateral cataract extractions on a woman in London. In 1775, surgeon George Chandler of London recounted that after cutting the cornea, Baron Wenzel would wait for the eye to finish rolling about before performing the capsulorhexis.[281] Philip Anthony Miller of Germany settled in Edinburgh by 1771 and introduced numerous ophthalmic tools adopted locally: an eyelid speculum used by Benjamin Bell, and a knife with a 90-degree turn that permitted either eye to be operated with the right hand, touted by Jonathan Wathen. George Borthwick of Edinburgh used both these tools. In 1769, John Goldwyer of Sarum (and later Salisbury) advertised that in London he had learned "the improved Operation on the Eye, for the Cataract, after the Method of Wensel and Hilmer."[282]

Although the traditional British surgeons dabbled with cataract extraction, oculists who traveled from the Continent continued to be the highest-volume performers of the technique—Baron Wenzel, Pellier, Miller, and Frederick William Jericho.

The first group of high-volume English oculists to master cataract extraction were the trio of Jonathan Wathen (c. 1728-1808), his student and subsequent partner James Ware (1756-1815), and Wathen's step-grandson Jonathan Wathen (Phipps) Waller (1769-1853). They performed extracapsular cataract extraction. As public

---

281 Leffler et al. "British Isles" 2021.

282 Leffler et al. "British Isles" 2021.

evidence of interest in cataract surgery appears for both Wathen and Ware at about the same time, it is unclear whether the teacher or student was the first to become interested in ophthalmology. Perhaps, their relationship was forged through this mutual interest. Ware, the student, actually was the first to write an ophthalmic treatise—his *Remarks on the Ophthalmy, Psorophthalmy and Purulent Eye* of 1780, which indicated at least some practical familiarity with cataract extraction. The mentor Wathen followed suit in 1785 with *A dissertation on the theory and cure of the cataract: in which the practice of extraction is supported.* Wathen had learned cataract extraction by experiments in animals and recommended the technique not only by his own experience over many years "but also by that of some others, who have practiced it in this country, in the course of the last twenty years."[283] This time frame corresponds with the arrival of Baron Wenzel to England in 1764. The junior members of the trio were less shy about explicitly acknowledging Wenzel as an important authority. In 1791, as his partnership with Wathen ended, Ware translated the *Traité de la cataracte* of Wenzel's son, which summarized the Baron's techniques. In addition, Ware indicated that "...he [Ware] has derived the most useful and important information, from the opportunities with which he was favoured of seeing the Baron operate, and from the remarks occasionally made by the Baron, on the different parts of his process." Likewise, in 1792, Phipps wrote that couching "has within these twenty years given place in this country to that of extraction, introduced by the late Baron de Wensel."[284]

In 1804, Phipps founded and served as the consulting and operating surgeon of the Royal Infirmary for the Diseases of the Eye in London, the first eye infirmary in the British Isles, and a surviving institution until 1872.

The competing surgeons John Cunningham Saunders and John Richard Farre, who in 1805 opened the London Infirmary for Curing Diseases of the Eye, which subsequently became the Moorfields Eye Hospital, reserved extraction for rare cases with exceptionally hard lenses. They generally preferred discission (division) of the lens. Farre explained: "...it is too well known how very limited the success of extraction in general practice has proved..."[285]

Some cataract innovations were proposed in the British Isles. In 1785, Benjamin Bell of Edinburgh proposed making the corneal incision for cataract extraction in the superior (rather than inferior) cornea. He was not aware of anyone doing this in humans and so he experimented with this technique in animals. When performing bilateral surgery, Wathen made the corneal incisions for both the left and right eyes before actually extracting either lens.[286]

---

283 Leffler et al. "British Isles" 2021.
284 Leffler et al. "British Isles" 2021.
285 Leffler et al. "British Isles" 2021.
286 Leffler et al. "British Isles" 2021.

Joseph Higgs, surgeon of Birmingham, proposed to John Theophilus Desaguliers (d. 1744) that couching of the lens might treat myopia. Higgs published the idea in 1755, but their conversation probably took place when Higgs was training in London in the mid-1720s.[287]

Conclusions

It is conceivable that cataract couching occurred in Roman Britain, based on the archaeological identification of Roman couching needles, and the mention of oculists there in ancient literature. Couching also could have been performed in the British Isles in the early Middle Ages and might correspond with stories of blindness miraculously cured by the clergy. If such eye surgeries did occur in the British Isles, their performance could have been negatively impacted by the Council of Tours in 1163 limiting clerical study of medicine, and by the expulsion of Jews from England in 1290. Manuscripts from continental Europe describing cataract couching were translated or copied in the British Isles throughout the late Middle Ages. However, there is actually no good evidence of cataract couching in the British Isles from the medieval period up until the Elizabethan era (beginning 1558). This absence of evidence is unlikely to reflect simply poor survival of records, given that we do have evidence of both nonsurgical ophthalmic care and nonophthalmic surgeries in the British Isles and of knowledge of medieval cataract couching from Southern Europe to Japan.

Beginning with the Elizabethan era, we have an explosion in evidence of cataract couching in the British Isles. We know the names of both surgeons performing and patients having the procedure. A new vernacular—oculist, cataract, and couching—took hold in the English language. This new procedure may have been reflected in Shakespeare's writing.

Cataract couching probably crossed the English Channel by the 1560s and arrived in Scotland in 1595, in Ireland in 1684, and in Anglo-America in 1751.

Throughout the 16th and 17th centuries, the primary institutions transmitting the knowledge of cataract surgery were families and mountebank troupes. British universities and hospitals do not seem to have played major roles. Beginning in the 1720s, cataract couching was performed by traditional surgeons in hospitals, though dedicated oculists still were probably the highest-volume eye surgeons.

Beginning in the 17th century, congenital cataract surgery provided an opportunity for the oculist to tout his special skills and for philosophers to explore the fundamental nature of visual perception. The 1727 couching of the 13-year-old Daniel Dolins by William Cheselden was said to have confirmed the theories of philosopher George Berkeley, but Dolins probably was not born blind, and did

---

287 Leffler et al. "British Isles" 2021.

not recover visual function. Moreover, Berkeley knew the Dolins family, and the case report uses language typical of Berkeley.

Planned cataract extraction moved into Britain very shortly after Daviel's exposition of the technique in Paris in 1752. Traditional surgeons in the British Isles did dabble with extraction, but still looked to high-volume dedicated oculists from the Continent as the authorities on the procedure. It is not until the 1780s that a group of English oculists led by Jonathan Wathen took over as the premier cataract-extracting group in England.

References

Allason-Jones L. Health care in the Roman north. *Britannia* 1999;30:133-146.

Baker PA. *Medical Care for the Roman Army on the Rhine, Danube and British Frontiers in the First, Second and Early Third Centuries AD*. Thesis University of Newcastle upon Tyne. 2000.

Banister R, Guillemeau J. *A Treatise of One Hundred and Thirteen Diseases of the Eyes*. New York: Da Capo; 1971.

Cheselden W. An account of some observations made by a young gentleman, who was born blind, or lost his sight so early, that he had no remembrance of ever having seen, and was couch'd between 13 and 14 years of age. By Mr. Will. Chesselden, F. R. S. Surgeon to Her Majesty, and to St. Thomas's Hospital. *Philos. Trans. R. Soc. Lond.* 1728;35(402):447-450.

Cheselden W. An explication of the instruments used, in a new operation on the eyes, by the same. *Philos. Trans. R. Soc. Lond.* 1728;35(402):451-452.

Dingwall HM. "To be insert in the mercury": Medical practitioners and the press in eighteenth-century Edinburgh. *Soc Hist Med.* 2000;13(1):23-44.

Duddell B. *A treatise of the diseases of the horny-coat of the eye, and the various kinds of cataracts. To which is prefix'd, a method, entirely new, of scarifying the eyes for several disorders…By Benedict Duddell, Surgeon and Oculist*. London: Clark; 1729: 174-176.

Gottfried RS. *Doctors and Medicine in Medieval England: 1340-1530*. Princeton: Princeton University Press; 1986.

Grapheus B (Grassus), Miranda-Garcia A, Gonzalez Fernandez-Corugedo S. *Benvenutus Grassus' On the well-proven art of the eye: Practica oculorum & De probatissima arte oculorum*. Synoptic Edition and Philological Studies. New York: Peter Lang; 2011.

James RR. *Studies in the History of Ophthalmology in England Prior to the Year 1800*. Cambridge: The University Press; 2013.

Leffler CT, Schwartz SG, Davenport B, et al. Enduring influence of Elizabethan ophthalmic texts of the 1580s: Bailey, Grassus, and Guillemeau. *Open Ophthalmol J.* 2014;8:12.

Leffler CT, Schwartz SG, Davenport B. Congenital cataract surgery during the early enlightenment period and the Stepkins oculists. *JAMA Ophthalmol.* 2014 Jul 1;132(7):883-884.

Leffler CT, Schwartz SG. A family of early English oculists (1600-1751), with a reappraisal of John Thomas Woolhouse (1664-1733/1734). *Ophthalmol Eye Dis.* 2017;9:1179172117732042.

Leffler CT, Schwartz SG. Glaucoma during the Enlightenment and early modern periods (1700-1849). In: Leffler CT (ed.), *The History of Glaucoma*. Amsterdam: Wayenborgh; 2020: 153-203.

Leffler CT, Klebanov A, Samara WA, et al. The history of cataract surgery: from couching to phacoemulsification. *Ann Transl Med.* 2020 Nov;8(22).

Leffler CT, Schwartz SG, Peterson E, et al. The first cataract surgeons in the British Isles. *Am J Ophthalmol*. 2021 Oct 1;230:75-122.

Leffler CT, Hogewind BF, Schwartz SG, et al. Jacques Daviel performed the first documented planned primary cataract extraction on Sep. 18, 1750. *Eye*. 2023 Dec 6:1-2.

Mullini R. "I Cornelius à Tilbourn": Hotchpotches, poisons, antidotes, and royal gifts. The career of a seventeenth-century London irregular physician. In: *Chlorophyll Killers: Pozioni, veleni, narcotici tra letteratura noir e scienza*. Fano: Aras; 2016: 119-148.

No author listed. Mr. Cheselden, a Surgeon of St. Thomas's Hospital, presented to her Royal Highness the Princess of Wales. *Daily Journal (London)*, March 14, 1727; (1923):1.

No author listed. *Detailed record for Harley 1585. Medical miscellany of a pharmacopeial compilation, including a herbal and bestiary illustrating the pharmocopeial properties of animals.* Available from: https://www.bl.uk/catalogues/illuminatedmanuscripts/record.asp?MSID=7970&CollID=8&NStart=1585 Accessed June 7, 2019.

No author listed. *Oxford, Bodleian Library, Ashmole 1462, folio 10r. The Mackinney Collection of Medieval Medical Illustrations*. Available from: https://dc.lib.unc.edu/cdm/ref/collection/mackinney/id/4045 Accessed June 7, 2019.

No author listed. Detailed record for Sloane 1975. *Medical and herbal collection, including Pseudo-Apuleius, Herbarius; Pseudo-Dioscorides, De herbis femininis (ff. 49v-73); Sextus Placitus, De medicina ex animalibus*. British Library. Available from: http://www.bl.uk/catalogues/illuminatedmanuscripts/record.asp?MSID=8792 Accessed June 7, 2019.

Phippy HR. *A biography of Jonathan Wathen Phipps/Waller. Eye-Surgeon to King George III*. Studley: Brewin; 2014.

Read W. *A short but exact account of all the diseases incident to the eyes, with the causes, symptoms and cures. Also practical observations…*London, [1709].

Schwartz SG, Leffler CT. Uses of the word "macula" in written English, 1400–present. *Surv Ophthalmol*. 2014;59(6):649-654.

Schwartz SG, Leffler CT. "Chevalier" John Taylor and His Descendants. In: *The History of Glaucoma*. Amsterdam: Wayenborg; 2020: 219.

Seabrooke R. *Seabrookes caueat: or His warning piece to all his loving country-men, to beware how they meddle with the eyes…*By Richard Seabrooke, practitioner in the art of the oculist. London: Edward All-de; 1620.

Talbot CH. *Medicine in Medieval England*. London: Oldbourne; 1967: 94,109,110,114.

2. John Thomas Woolhouse (1664–1733/4) and His Family of Oculists (1600–1751)

Christopher T. Leffler, MD, MPH
Stephen G. Schwartz, MD, MBA

Introduction

Ophthalmology in Northern Europe progressed substantially from the Elizabethan era through the mid-1700s. Ophthalmic healing during this period was a craft handed down from generation to generation within families. One such family was that of John Thomas Woolhouse (1664–1733/4) of England. He wrote that he was one of four generations of fathers and sons who practiced eye surgery. Historians have known a little about his oculist father, Thomas Woolhouse (1628–1688). With today's digital resources and databases, it is possible to tell the stories of at least eight oculists in his family over five generations, spanning 1600 to 1751 (Fig. 1).[1]

Mr. Atwood of Worcestershire

The oculist patriarch of the family was one Mr. Atwood of Worcestershire.[2] Little is known about him, except that his daughter Judith married John Stepkins in Wolverley parish in 1625.[3] Later Atwood oculists can be identified, though whether they are related to the Woolhouse family is unknown. In 1655, Mr. Atwood, "an oculist of good fame" treated one Mr. Alsop of Derbyshire.[4] Author Samuel Johnson remembered that in 1711: "... my mother carried me to Trysul, to consult Dr. [Thomas] Atwood, an oculist of Worcester."[5] Trysull is about 12 miles from Wolverley.

John Stepkins (c. 1600–1652)

Atwood's son-in-law John Stepkins was consistently described as an eminent oculist. Stepkins had several medical influences. In 1606, his maternal uncle John Bramston (1577–1654) married Bridget, the daughter of Richard Moundeford (1550–1630), a prominent London physician.[6] This connection sounds distant, but the families must have been close. When Stepkins' wife died, he needed a guardian for his daughter Theodosia (known later as Lady Ivy), and he placed her with Mrs.

---

1 Parish Register. Halstead, Essex, 1664; Marriage of Judeth Attwood ... 1625.

2 Leffler 2014, p. 883.

3 Robinson 1903, p. 107.

4 Rutland 1889, pp. 5–347.

5 Boswell 1868, p. 318.

6 Moore 2004.

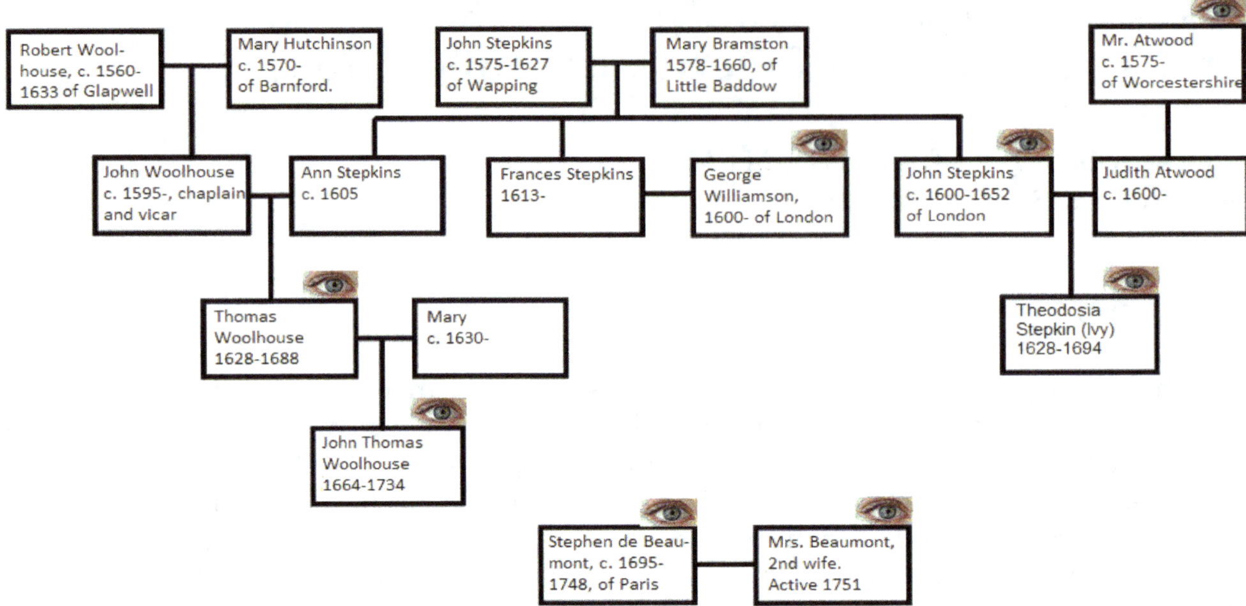

Fig. 1. Family tree of the Stepkins and Woolhouse oculists. Stephen de Beaumont was the nephew of John Thomas Woolhouse.

Moundeford.[7] Mrs. Moundeford herself sometimes treated the sick. In 1615, when an oculist was unsuccessful in treating a girl with a disorder of the eyes, Mrs. Moundeford was called upon to nurse her back to health.[8]

But it was Stepkins' father-in-law who taught him the most: Stepkins "maried to Mrs. [Judith] Atwood, in Worcestershire, daughter of a very famous oculist, [of] whome this John learned much of his skill, tho' he improved by practice extreamly."[9]

Stepkins was known for a variety of eye waters, and for performing congenital cataract surgery.[10] Congenital cataract surgery had been performed in about 1000 AD by Ammaar ibn Alii Mawṣilii of Cairo, who couched a 30-year-old man from Kurdistan with a congenital cataract.[11] (For this case, Ammar did not use the hollow needle he later devised to extract soft cataracts by suction.) Still, Stepkins performed the earliest congenital cataract surgery of which we are aware in England, as described by Robert Boyle:

> The bare prospect of this magnificent Fabric of the Universe, furnished and adorned with such strange variety of curious and useful Creatures, would, suffice to transport us both with Wonder and Joy, if their Commonness did not hinder their Operations.

---

7 Jenkins 1949, pp. 57–80.

8 Pelling 2004.

9 Bramston 1845, pp. 17–19.

10 Leffler 2014, p. 883.

11 'Ammār ibn 'Alī Mawṣilī 1937, pp. 33–57.

74

Of which Truth Mr Stepkins, the famous Oculist, did not long since supply us with a memorable Instance: For (as both himself and an Illustrious Person that was present at the Cure informed me) a Maid of about Eighteen years of Age, having by a couple of Cataracts, that she brought with her into the World, lived absolutely blind from the moment of her Birth; being brought to the free Use of her Eyes, was so ravished at the surprising spectacle of so many and various Objects, as presented themselves to her unacquainted Sight, that almost everything she saw transported her with such admiration and delight, that she was in danger to lose the eyes of her Mind by those of her Body, and expound that Mystical Arabian Proverb, which advises, To shut the Windows, that the House may be Light.[12]

According to Boyle, the treatment was "a manual operation" performed "by my Ingenious Acquaintance, Mr. Stepkins." Stepkins died and was buried on May 19, 1652 at St Mary's Whitechapel church in London.[13]

George Williamson (1600–After 1663)

George Williamson married John Stepkins' sister Frances in 1633.[14] Stepkins lodged with Williamson at the time of his death in 1652.[15] A physician recorded that his 87-year-old father-in-law, David Tryme, from Wookey, near Bath, was unsuccessfully operated on by Williamson in 1663. The inflammation in the nonoperated eye could suggest sympathetic ophthalmia:

For, contrary to Dr. [Dawbeney] Turbervile's Advice, (who counselled him to stay till he had been quite blind, when the Cataracts would have been ripe ...). He hearing of one in London, in whose House Stephkin, the famous Occulist, formerly lodged (Father to my Lady Ivy, who also professed Eye-mending). This Fellow having seen Mr. Stephkin often perform that Operation, thought himself very able to do it, and set up for himself, (when his Lodger was dead,) and had a considerable Reputation for this Operation. This old Gentleman [Tryme] made a London-Journey at 87 Years of Age, or more; submits to this Fellow's Cure; who without any kind of Preparation, of bleeding, or purging ... performed the Operation ... This brought such a Flux of Humours first to that Eye, (for he had Couched but one) then to the other, afterwards to the whole Head ... but caused him to lead a miserable Life the remainder of his Days ... about a Year and some Months.[16]

---

12 Boyle 1663, pp. 3, 75.

13 Stepkins 1651; Ivie 1654; London ... Marriages 1538–1812.

14 Marriage of Fran Stepkin ... 1538–1850.

15 Stepkins 1651.

16 Pierce 1697, pp. 169–170.

Theodosia Stepkins (Lady Ivy, 1628–1695)

Stepkins had a daughter named Theodosia, who through her marriage later became known as Lady Ivy (1628–1695).[17] When she was a child, her mother died sometime after the last sibling was born in 1631. Therefore, her father placed her in the London home of Mrs. Moundeford, as noted above.[18]

Theodosia was notorious in her day, and has been remembered for centuries, for several unfortunate episodes. In the early 1650s, she demanded alimony from her husband, Thomas Ivy.[19] Theodosia made allegations of assault, infidelity, and infection with venereal disease, and Thomas Ivy made counterclaims of deceit, profligacy, murder of a chambermaid by poisoning, and conspiracy to murder him. Nonetheless, they reconciled in 1660, and Theodosia became "Lady Ivy" when her husband was knighted in 1661.[20] When she sustained property losses in the Wapping (London) fire of 1682, she was hailed "... for her great pitty and Charity."[21]

In 1684, leases Lady Ivy claimed established her ownership of property near Wapping were determined to be forgeries in a civil case.[22] However, in the 1686 criminal trial for forgery, which was a capital offense, Lady Ivy was acquitted.[23]

In her day Lady Ivy was also well known as an oculist. Unlike her father, her reputation as a healer appears to have been mixed. Lady Ivy, like her father, was known for applying eye waters.[24] We have no evidence that she performed cataract couching.

Thomas Woolhouse (1628–1688)

A chaplain named John Woolhouse joined this family of oculists by marrying John Stepkins' sister Ann in London in 1627.[25] John Woolhouse was a chaplain to the East India Company from 1619 until the year of his marriage. He was "ejected" as the Vicar of West Mersey, Essex in 1642, during the English Civil War.[26] It seems that the minister never pursued a medical career. His oculist son Thomas Woolhouse wrote in 1675: "My father, being the first minister in Essex ... that was plundered

---

17 Leffler 2014, p. 883.

18 Jenkins 1949, pp. 57–80.

19 Jenkins 1949, pp. 57–80; Ivie 1654; Neale 1929, pp. 1–100.

20 Jenkins 1949, pp. 57–80.

21 Quote from: Sad and lamentable news ... 1682, p. 4; also: A more full ... 1682, p. 2.

22 Jenkins 1949, pp. 57–80; Mossam 1696, pp. 1–80.

23 Jenkins 1949, pp. 57–80; Neale 1929, pp. 1–100.

24 Leffler 2014, p. 883.

25 Marriage of Ann Stepkin ... 1538–1850.

26 Venn 1927, p. 462.

of any person whatsoever in Essex for his loyalty, was made incapable of giving me any other learning than reading the Bible ...”[27] Thomas Woolhouse entered the Colchester School in Essex in 1641 at age 13.[28]

Thomas Woolhouse served as the Page of the Presence (personal attendant) to King Charles II from March 19, 1673/4 until the king's death in 1685.[29] On May 11, 1686, the appointment was renewed by the king's brother and successor James II until Woolhouse's death.[30] According to his son, this royal service was in the capacity of an oculist. Thomas Woolhouse travelled to France to successfully treat Henry Howard (1655–1701), the seventh Duke of Norfolk, who had a “violent Ophthalmy and Defluxion on his Eyes.”[31] The Duke went to France on March 24, 1688.[32] Woolhouse died and was buried on May 30, 1688.[33]

John Thomas Woolhouse (1664–1733/4)

John Thomas Woolhouse was born in Halstead, Essex, and was baptized at St. Andrew's church on December 23, 1664.[34] In 1675, when he was 11 years old, his father wrote to the royal secretary:

> As it is your favour to receive my son into your service we are ready to receive your commands ... Though he has not that complaisant humour the City brings forth, being always bred near Colchester till these two years, I hope you will find more genius in him to receive your commands than it is expedient to express, he being my son. He has had the experience of the want of learning ... I have endeavoured to make him sensible thereby to quicken up his genius not to lose any opportunity.[35]

John Thomas Woolhouse claimed that he couched cataracts at age 13,[36] presumably as an apprentice to his father. On April 26, 1681, a warrant was issued for him to have the first vacancy as Page of the Presence to Charles II,[37] a position occupied by his father. Woolhouse matriculated at Trinity College in Cambridge in 1684 and

---

27 Blackburne 1907, p. 4.

28 Acland 1897, p. 40.

29 Woolhouse, Thomas 1660–1901.

30 Woolhouse, Thomas, Royal Archives, 1660–1901; Will of Thomas Woolhouse 1688.

31 Woolhouse 1701.

32 Lee 1891, p. 33.

33 Burial of Thomas Woolhouse 1688.

34 Parish Register. Halstead, Essex. St Andrew's church. December 23, 1664. John, son of Thomas Wolhouse and Mary. www.freereg.org.uk

35 Blackburne 1907, p. 4.

36 Hirschberg 1984, vol. 3, pp. 5–369; Woolhouse 1721, pp. 4–66.

37 Woolhouse, “Page of the presence to Charles II. 26 Apl. 1681.”

graduated in 1686–1687.[38] He studied eye surgery at Oxford.[39] He converted to Catholicism, and was therefore "disinherited by his father."[39 40] Upon his father's death, it seems that he replaced his father as oculist to James II (who was exiled in December 1688 with the Glorious Revolution).

John Thomas Woolhouse left England after the revolution. In 1724, he wrote that he left due to the unhealthful London air: "the sealcoal air of London gave me a consumption in my youth which has been the chief cause of my fixing in this city [Paris]."[34] But in 1698, he had written that he left to follow James II into exile: "Ever since the King my Master left England I have constantly attended him ... as well in Ireland as in France, excepting about three years' time ... to study at Paris, Avignon, Montpellier, Pisa and Rome, and the late eight months I spent at Mons, Brussels, Maastricht, Aix la Chapelle, Liége, Cologne, etc., in the exercise of my profession of oculist ..."[39]

In Paris, Woolhouse became the surgeon at the Hôpital des Quinze-Vingts. He wrote in 1696 that he was the oculist to the exiled James II. He wrote that he could "give sight to those that are blind of cataracts, gutta serenas, pearls ..." In 1698, Woolhouse requested to return to "my native country" given "my desire of marrying in England." He promised not to make trouble with the state, and "to treat all blind and sore-eyed curable poor people gratis." He was told that his Catholicism and service to James II would make his return highly unlikely.[40]

We could not find any record of a wife or children for Woolhouse. Perhaps, he ultimately married in France, given that he referred to Stephen de Beaumont of France as his nephew.

The ophthalmic historian Julius Hirschberg reported that Woolhouse served as the oculist to William III, who died in 1702.[41] Such service would be highly unlikely, as Woolhouse's Catholicism and service to the exiled James II prevented him from even returning to England. In fact, Woolhouse was appointed oculist to James III by royal warrant on September 20, 1707.[42] At this time, James III lived in exile in France, but claimed the throne of England as the son of James II. Known in England as "the Pretender," James III was evicted from France in 1713.

Woolhouse knew about his oculist heritage. He wrote that he was one of four generations of fathers and sons who were oculists,[43] that his family had many women oculists, and specifically mentioned Stepkins, Lady Ivy,[44] and his father.

---

38 Venn 1927, p. 462.

39 Hirschberg 1984, vol. 3, pp. 5–369; Woolhouse, October 1707, pp. 299–305.

40 Calendar of the Manuscripts of the Marquis of Bath, 1908, pp. 290–295.

41 Hirschberg 1984, vol. 3, pp. 5–369.

42 Calendar of the Stuart Papers belonging to His Majesty the King, 1902, p. 215.

43 James 1934.

44 Woolhouse March 1701; Woolhouse, October 1707, p. 299; Woolhouse March 1696, p. 53.

Woolhouse's reputation extended to Moscow.[45] In fact, Woolhouse demonstrated the cataract operation for Peter the Great in Paris in 1717, and the Tsar requested that Woolhouse teach a Russian student.[46]

The Private Ophthalmology Course

Woolhouse was teaching ophthalmology by about 1693. At times, his classes held 12 students from throughout Europe.[47] He was still teaching as of 1725. His lectures were at least partly in French.[48]

The duration of training may have varied. One student, Christophe LeCerf, wrote "Woolhouse is the only one in Europe who can give within one month a complete course on two hundred eye diseases with patient demonstrations and lectures. He lets his pupils operate as much as they wish to."[49] The lecture series of 1721 lasted approximately 3 months.[50] Johannes Zacharias Platner, MD (1694–1747) and another prominent German student, Burkard David Mauchart (1696–1751), studied for 9 months in 1720.[51]

Proponents and detractors agreed that the training provided extensive hands-on experience. The English student, Benedict Duddell (c. 1695–c. 1765), stated: "… I have examin'd above a hundred blind in a Day at Paris, under Mr. Woolhouse in the Hospital of the Blind."[52] On the other hand, the French oculist Charles de Saint-Yves (1667–1736) wrote: "in Paris the eyes of poor people are sacrificed with impunity and without caution in order to have some material for apprentices who practice this operation for the first few months."[53]

The Students of Woolhouse

Woolhouse's best-known students were Platner, Mauchart, and Duddell.[54] Duddell studied with Woolhouse in 1718,[55] and then settled in Hammersmith, near London. In 1736, Duddell offered one of the earliest descriptions of keratoconus.[56]

45 Hirschberg 1984, vol. 3.
46 Gerebtzoff 1862, p. 298.
47 James 1934.
48 Woolhouse 1745.
49 Hirschberg 1984, vol. 3.
50 Woolhouse 1721.
51 Hirschberg 1984, vol. 3.
52 Duddell 1729.
53 Hirschberg 1984, vol. 3.
54 Wyman 1992, p. 412.
55 Duddell 1729.
56 Grzybowski 2013, p. 140.

Woolhouse had kept his method of conjunctival scarification with beards of barley a secret, but one time Woolhouse got drunk, and Mauchart wheedled the secret out of him. Mauchart "wrote an extensive manuscript about this course which he took with him and used occasionally in his later publications." Mauchart hoped after his stay in Paris to study in Leiden, but the border was closed due to the bubonic plague. He eventually became a professor in Tübingen, and died of an asthma attack in 1751, at the age of 55.[57] Platner became a professor at Leipzig, and rose to be the dean, before dying of an asthma attack at age 53.

We know of Woolhouse's teachings from his journal articles, and also from the books published by his students. LeCerf assembled letters and manuscripts of Woolhouse written between 1707 and 1716, and published them in French in 1717.[58]

Highlights of a manuscript containing notes from Woolhouse's 1721 lecture series recorded by a student were published in 1934. The manuscript from the Royal Society of Medicine is entitled: "A Treatise of ye Cataract & Glaucoma. Dictated by Mons. Woolhouse, Occulist to ye French King, begun April 29, 1721."[59] We obtained this manuscript from the Royal Society of Medicine. Quotations from the 1721 lecture notes in our book use modern spellings.

Woolhouse's teachings on cataract and glaucoma were published in 1745 by an anonymous student who made a written record of the lectures given in Paris "above twenty years ago."[60] The 1745 text includes at least some of the same anecdotes and teachings from the 1721 lecture notes.

The most extensive reviews of Woolhouse's life and contributions were prepared by Hirschberg, and by R. R. James in 1934.

Woolhouse's contributions with respect to hydrophthalmia, glaucoma, lensectomy (even before Daviel), and synechiolysis were covered in previous chapters. Before 1705, he emphasized hydrophthalmia, a condition of excess ocular tension treated with paracentesis. After 1705, he emphasized glaucoma in response to the new theory of the nature of cataract. He stated that glaucoma involved a palpably hard eye. Finally, after 1715, he acknowledged that couching was typically displacing the crystalline lens (though he still refused to call this a cataract). He would extract the lens if it happened to enter the anterior chamber during couching.

Woolhouse was known for several advances not directly related to glaucoma. He was a pioneer with respect to congenital cataract surgery.[61] As early as 1698, he

---

57 Hirschberg 1984, vol. 4.

58 Woolhouse, LeCerf 1717.

59 James 1934; Woolhouse 1721.

60 Woolhouse 1745.

61 Leffler 2014.

wrote that he had "cured those that have been born blind."[62] He had performed 36 documented congenital cataract surgeries by 1721, the youngest in a patient 18 months of age.[63] In several other areas, Woolhouse was a pioneer.

Dacryocystectomy

Woolhouse's method of treating dacryocystitis involved extirpation of the lacrimal gland, cautery of the ethmoid bone, and placement of a golden tubule leading into the lacrimal fossa. Placement of the tubule had been done previously by Heister. Hirschberg noted Duddell's account that the ancients were not intending to remove the lacrimal sac, and their cauterization therefore accomplished this inconsistently or incompletely.[64] In fact, we found this statement in the manuscript of Woolhouse's 1721 lectures. Hirschberg credits Woolhouse with being the first author to recommend dacryocystectomy, a treatment which was standard for recalcitrant dacryocystitis until the invention of dacryocystorhinostomy in 1904, and which can still be used when the latter procedure is inappropriate.[65] Historians have known of Woolhouse's method only because it was described by Platner and by Duddell. Woolhouse's words on the matter have never been published. We found the following passage in Woolhouse's 1721 lecture manuscript:

> There is a particular case in ye hernia of ye lacrimal sac become varicose, and mightily distended and hard, drawing after it ye entire nasal conduit outwards, which must be extirpated entirely all at once, and cauterized likewise, which to prevent a great effusion of blood, and which to hinder ye distortion of ye eyelids which a great suppuration would infallibly produce.

Return to England

Woolhouse's letters place him in Paris through July 1730, after which time he returned to England. If he practiced as an oculist upon his return, he did not leave any records that we could identify. Woolhouse died on January 26, 1733 (1734 by the New Style calendar).[66]

---

62 Calendar of the Manuscripts of the Marquis of Bath 1908, p. 290.

63 Woolhouse 1721.

64 Hirschberg 1984, vol. 3.

65 Matayoshi 2004.

66 James 1934.

Stephen de Beaumont

In England, his nephew Stephen de Beaumont, MD (d. 1748)[67] continued the family tradition as an oculist. Beaumont was a native of France, and was in Provence in about 1718. The first indication that he performed some medical procedures comes from a letter by Woolhouse in 1728: "My son Beaumont does the operation well & I've taken several ounces of this remedy, & do believe it sav'd myself in a great fluxion I had on my breast." In 1729, Beaumont's wife delivered her first child, but both mother and child died, the former after a period of illness.[68] Woolhouse's obituary in January 1734 noted he "Last week died at his nephew's Mr. Beaumont, in St. Martin's-lane."[69] Beaumont was executor of his estate, and inherited his property.[70] Beaumont had begun practicing as an oculist by 1736: "Mr. Beaumont, a celebrated Occulist, couch'd in the French Hospital several Pensioners of that House, who all recover'd their Sight soon after, tho' some of them were upwards of seventy."[71]

Beaumont was strongly suspected of being a Jacobite sympathizer. In 1738, he was charged with speaking treasonous words—specifically drinking to the health of the Pretender (James III).[72] In 1739, came the dramatic news:

> Dr. Beaumont, an eminent French Oculist in St. Martin's-lane, was taken into Custody of his Majesty's Messengers ... it's given out that the former is charg'd with aiding and assisting Mr. George Kelly in his Escape from the Tower, and for corresponding with him since at Avignon.—*Heaven defend us from a Plot.*[73]

Kelly (d. 1750), an Irish clergyman, had been imprisoned in the Tower of London after his arrest in 1722 for a pro-Jacobite conspiracy, but had escaped to France in 1736. Beaumont was released on bail.

We do not know what happened with either charge, but Beaumont appears to have found social outlets in which he was accepted. He became a leader in the Masons by 1738.[74] As freemasonry was essentially a British export, Beaumont permitted the establishment of a lodge in Frankfurt.[75] In 1742, he proposed that the portrait of Frederick, Prince of Wales, be hung in the London masonic lodge.[76] Beaumont was

---

67 Anderson 1738, p. 139.

68 James 1934.

69 Last week died ... January 28, 1734.

70 James 1934.

71 Quote from: On Tuesday last Mr. Beaumont ... June 10, 1736. Also: On Monday last Mr. Beaumont ... June 4, 1736.

72 Rex v Stephen BEAUMONT ... 1738; Osborne 1749, p. 21.

73 Quote from: Dr. Beaumont, an eminent French Oculist in St. Martin's-lane ... January 6–9, 1739. Also see: An Oculist in St. Martin's Lane ... January 13, 1739.

74 Anderson 1738; Pocket companion ... 1754.

75 Gould 1906.

76 At a full Lodge of Free-Masons ... February 26, 1742.

repaid by being named the oculist to the Prince of Wales.[77] It might seem odd that the prince would include in his court an oculist ostensibly devoted to the overthrow of his father, King George II. However, the prince and his father were estranged, and the prince established an opposition court.

Beaumont died in 1748.[78] In 1751, his widow advertised "her late Husband's most excellent Collyrium, or Eye-Water, for curing Inflammations in the Eyes, and strengthening Weak Sight."[79] Thus ends the known record of the five generations of oculists in the Stepkins and Woolhouse family.

Conclusions

John Thomas Woolhouse was an eye surgeon in a family of five generations of English oculists. He was an early adopter of paracentesis for hydrophthalmia, a condition of excess ocular tension. In response to the new theory that a cataract was an opacity of the crystalline lens, he focused attention on the term *glaucoma*, which had been applied to disorders of the lens by the ancients. He observed that swelling of the lens could lead to palpable hardness of the eye, which, due to its origin with the lens, he termed *glaucoma*. It is partly because of Woolhouse that *glaucoma*, which initially suggested a lens disorder, has come to describe an optic neuropathy for which elevated intraocular pressure is a risk factor. Woolhouse also appreciated that the soft eye was unlikely to recover vision. Woolhouse was also a pioneer with respect to surgery for synechiolysis, dacryocystectomy, and congenital cataracts.

Acknowledgments

The authors would like to thank Damaris Kuzminski, an independent genealogic researcher, who figured out how the family trees of Stepkins and Woolhouse connected, and who found important historical documents, such as John Thomas Woolhouse's baptismal record.

References

A few days ago died Dr. Beaumont, Oculist to his Royal Highness the Prince of Wales. Penny London Post or The Morning Advertiser (London, England), November 7–9, 1748; Issue 1023.

A more full and exact account of that most dreadful fire which happened at Wapping on Sunday night the nineteenth of this instant Novemb. London: Printed by D. Mallet; 1682:2.

---

77 An account of the proceedings, 1744; An account of the proceedings, 1747; A few days ago died Dr. Beaumont November 7–9, 1748.

78 A few days ago died Dr. Beaumont ... November 7–9, 1748.

79 Beaumont, August 13, 1751.

Acland CL, Round JH. Register of the Scholars Admitted to Colchester School, 1637–1740. Colchester: Wiles & Son; 1897:40.

'Ammār ibn 'Alī Mawṣilī, Meyerhof M. Las Operaciones de catarata de 'Ammar ibn 'Ali al-Mawsili. Barcelona: Laboratories del Norte de Espana; 1937:33–57.

An account of the proceedings of the governors of St. George's hospital near Hyde-Park-Corner, from its first institution, October the nineteenth 1733 to the twenty-eighth of December 1743. St. George's Hospital. London; 1744:3.

An account of the proceedings of the governors of St. George's hospital near Hyde-Park-Corner, from its first institution, October the nineteenth 1733 to the thirty-first of December 1746. St. George's Hospital. London; 1747:3.

Anderson J. The New Book of Constitutions of the Antient and Honourable Fraternity of Free and Accepted Masons. London: Ward; 1738:139.

An Oculist in St. Martin's Lane...was taken into Custody. Common Sense or The Englishman's Journal (London, England), Saturday, January 13, 1739; Issue 102.

At a full Lodge of Free-Masons...Dr. Beaumont. Daily Post (London, England), Friday, February 26, 1742; Issue 7013.

Beaumont. The Widow of the Late Dr. Beaumont. General Advertiser (1744) (London, England), Tuesday, August 13, 1751; Issue 5246.

Blackburne DFH. Thomas Woollhouse to Williamson. Calendar of State Papers, Domestic Series, March 1st, 1675, to February 29th, 1676. London: Mackie and Co.; 1907:4.

Boswell J, Johnson S. The Life of Samuel Johnson, LL.D. London: Bell & Daldy; 1868:318.

Boyle R. Some considerations touching the vsefulnesse of experimental naturall philosophy propos'd in familiar discourses to a friend, by way of invitation to the study of it. Oxford: Printed by Hen. Hall for Ric. Davis; 1663:3–75.

Bramston J. The Autobiography of Sir John Bramston. London, England: Camden Society; 1845:17–19.

Burial of Thomas Woolhouse. May 30, 1688. St. Margaret. Westminster Burials Transcription. Findmypast.com.

Calendar of the Manuscripts of the Marquis of Bath. Vol. III. Hereford: Anthony Brothers Ltd; 1908:290–295.

Calendar of the Stuart Papers belonging to His Majesty the King. Vol. I. London: Mackie &Co; 1902:215.

Dr. Beaumont, an eminent French Oculist in St. Martin's-lane, was taken into Custody. London Evening Post (London, England), January 6, 1739–January 9, 1739; Issue 1740.

Duddell B. A Treatise of the Diseases of the Horny-Coat of the Eye, and the Various Kinds of Cataracts. London: John Clark; 1729:iv–230.

Gerebtzoff M. History of Civilization in Russia. Reviewed in: British Foreign Medical Review. London: John Churchill; October 1862:298.

Gould RF. A Library of Freemasonry: Comprising Its History, Antiquities, Symbols, Constitutions, Customs, Etc. Philadelphia: John C. Yorston; 1906:37.

Grzybowski A, McGhee CN. The early history of keratoconus prior to Nottingham's landmark 1854 treatise on conical cornea: a review. Clin Exp Optometry. 2013;96(2):140–145.

Hirschberg J, Blodi FC. The History of Ophthalmology, Vol. 3. The Renaissance of Ophthalmology in the Eighteenth Century (Part One). Bonn: J. P. Wayenborgh Verlag; 1984:5–369.

Hirschberg J, Blodi FC. The History of Ophthalmology, Vol. 4. The Renaissance of Ophthalmology in the Eighteenth Century (Part Two). Bonn: J. P. Wayenborgh Verlag; 1984:16–47.

Ivie T. Alimony arraign'd, or The remonstrance and humble appeal of Thomas Ivie Esq...London; 1654.

James RR. Woolhouse (1666--1733-4). Br J Ophthalmol. 1934;18(4):193–217.

Jenkins E. Six Criminal Women. New York: Duell, Sloan and Pearce; 1949:57–80.

Last week died at his nephew's Mr. Beaumont...John-Thomas Woolhouse. Penny London Post (London, England), Monday, January 28, 1734; Issue 67.

Lee S (ed.). Dictionary of National Biography, Vol. 28. New York: MacMillan and Co; 1891:33.

Leffler CT, Schwartz SG, Davenport B. Congenital cataract surgery during the early enlightenment period and the Stepkins oculists. JAMA Ophthalmol. 2014;132(7):883–884.

London, England, Church of England Baptisms, Marriages and Burials, 1538–1812 for John Stepkins. Tower Hamlets St Mary, Whitechapel 1644–1664. www.ancestry.com

Marriage of Ann Stepkin and John Woolhouse. 1627. St. Olave Silver Street. Boyd's marriage indexes, 1538–1850. Findmypast.com.

Marriage of Fran Stepkin and George Williamson. Faculty Office Marriage Licenses. England, Boyd's Marriage Indexes, 1538–1850. Search.findmypast.com

Marriage of Judeth Attwood and John Stepkin. 27 August 1625. Wolverley. ancestry.com. England, Select Marriages, 1538–1973. Provo, UT, USA.

Matayoshi S, Van Baak A, Cozac A, Sardinha M, Dias Fernandes JBV, da Mota Moura E. Dacryocystectomy: indications and results. Orbit. 2004;23:169–173.

Moore N, 'Moundeford, Thomas (1550–1630)', rev. Patrick Wallis, Oxford Dictionary of National Biography, Oxford University Press; 2004.

Mossam E. The famous tryal in B.R. between Thomas Neale, Esq. and the late Lady Theadosia Ivy the 4th of June, 1684...with a pamphlet heretofore writ... by Sir Thomas Ivy. 1696:1–80.

Neale (Thomas), Theodosia Ivie, George Jeffreys. The Lady Ivie's Trial for Great Part of Shadwell...before Lord Chief Justice Jeffreys in 1684. Edited by John C. Fox. Clarendon Press: Oxford; 1929:1–100.

On Monday last Mr. Beaumont, a famous Oculist. Daily Post (London), June 4, 1736; Issue 5219.

On Tuesday last Mr. Beaumont, a celebrated Occulist, couch'd in the French Hospital several Pensioners. Old Whig or The Consistent Protestant (London), June 10, 1736; Issue 66.

Osborne T. A catalogue of thirty thousand volumes, (with the Prices printed) of Several libraries...London; 1749:21.

Parish Register. Halstead, Essex. St Andrew's church. December 23, 1664. John, son of Thomas Wolhouse and Mary. www.freereg.org.uk

Pelling M, White F. 'BOWNE, Robert', in Physicians and Irregular Medical Practitioners in London 1550–1640 Database (London, 2004), British History Online. www.british-history.ac.uk

Pierce R. Bath memoirs: or, observations in three and forty years practice...Bristol: Hammond; 1697:169–170.

Rex v Stephen BEAUMONT for drinking the Pretender's health on 10 June, 11 Geo II (1738): Middlesex sessions. UK National Archives. 1738. Manuscript Number TS 11/424.

Robinson J. The Attwood Family, with Historic Notes & Pedigrees. Sunderland: Hills & Company; 1903:107.

Rutland C. The Manuscripts of His Grace the Duke of Rutland, K.G., Preserved at Belvoir Castle. Vol. II. London: Her Majesty's Stationery Office; 1889:5–347.

Sad and lamentable news from VVapping...a most horrible and dreadful fire, which happened on Sunday the 19th. of Nov. 1682...the great losses of...the Lady Ivy. London: Clarke; 1682:4.

Stepkins J. Will of John Stepkin or Stepkins of Wapping, Middlesex. 1651. National Archives of the UK. discovery.nationalarchives.gov.uk

The pocket companion and history of free-masons, containing their origine, progress, and present state: an abstract of their laws, constitutions, customs. London: J. Scott; 1754:189.

Venn J, Venn JA. Alumni Cantabrigienses; A Biographical List of All Known Students, Graduates and Holders of Office at the University of Cambridge, from the Earliest Times to 1900. Part 1. Volume 4. London: Cambridge University Press; 1927:462.

Woolhouse J. "Page of the presence to Charles II. 26 Apl. 1681". The Royal Archives. Royal Household Staff-1526-1924. Royal Household Index 1660–1901. Findmypast.co.uk

Woolhouse JT. Mr. Woolhouse, Gentil-homme Anglois. Mercure Galant. Paris: Chez Michel Brunet; March 1696:53–57. Gallica.bnf.fr

Woolhouse JT. Thomas Woolhouse, Esq...related to the late Famous Oculist, my Lady Ivy Post Man and the Historical Account (London, England), March 27–19, 1701; Issue 817.

Woolhouse JT. Le Roy d'Angleterre, scachant qu'il y a des personnes a Paris qui se dissent Oculistes. Mercure Galant. Paris: Chez Michel Brunet; October 1707:299–305. Gallica.bnf.fr

Woolhouse JT. A Treatise of ye Cataract & Glaucoma. Royal Society of Medicine Manuscript; 1721:4–66.

Woolhouse JT. A Treatise of the Cataract and Glaucoma: In Which the Specific Distinctions of Those Two Diseases, and the Existence of Membranous Cataracts, are Clearly Demonstrated...as Taken from Him in Writing, by One of His Pupils. London: Cooper; 1745:3–116.

"Woolhouse, Thomas. Page of the presence...reappointed James 1st... dead by 1688". The Royal Archives. Royal Household Staff 1526–1924. Volume: Royal Household Index, 1660–1901. Findmypast.co.uk.

Woolhouse T. Will of Thomas Woolhouse, Page of the Present Chamber to His Majesty of Saint Margaret Westminster, Middlesex. June 1688. National Archives of the UK. discovery.nationalarchives.gov.uk

Woolhouse JT, LeCerf C. Dissertations scavantes et critiques de monsieur de Woolhouse sur la cataracte et le glaucoma. Offenbach sur le Main: Bonaventure; 1717:21–299. Biusante.parisdescartes.fr

Wyman AL. Benedict Duddell: pioneer oculist of the 18th century. J Royal Soc Med. 1992;85:412–415.

3. "Chevalier" John Taylor and His Descendants

Stephen G. Schwartz, MD, MBA
Christopher T. Leffler, MD, MPH

Introduction

Prior to the 19th century, many European oculists lacked academic surgical training, and many practiced as itinerant surgeons, with associated negative connotations.[1] Perhaps the most famous, or infamous, of these was the physician John Taylor. Taylor was of common birth but called himself "Chevalier," French for "knight" (equivalent to the Italian "Cavaliere," the Spanish "Caballero," and the German "Ritter"). His professional legacy is controversial, and he was accused of charlatanism by many of his contemporaries and by many historians. His personal legacy is more favorable. His son John was a respected oculist, whose two sons, John and Jeremiah, also practiced honorably. Their lives illustrate ophthalmic care in 18th- and 19th-century Europe.[2]

Chevalier John Taylor (1703–1772)

John Taylor was born in Norwich circa 1703, a son of a surgeon also named John (Fig. 1). Taylor's grandson John subsequently wrote: "The chevalier, whom I was too young to remember, was, I have always heard, a tall, handsome man, and a great favourite with the ladies. He was much addicted to splendour in dress, and to an expensive style of domestic expenditure ..."[3]

Taylor was trained by William Cheselden (1688–1752) in London. He started as an oculist and general surgeon in Norwich, but began practicing as an itinerant in Britain in 1727, and throughout Europe in 1734. Taylor claimed to hold a university faculty position at Avignon,[4] which has been disputed.[5] Taylor did earn medical degrees from Basel, Reims, Liège, and Cologne in 1734–1735, although these have been criticized as "honorary foreign degrees."[6]

Taylor met Jacques Daviel (1693–1762) in Marseille in 1734 and claimed to have introduced him to eye surgery,[7–9] which has been disputed.[10] Nevertheless, Daviel did for a time also practice as an itinerant oculist,[8] perhaps influenced by Taylor. Daviel ultimately introduced planned cataract extractions, which Taylor attempted but never fully accepted.[11]

Taylor was appointed Royal Oculist to King George II in 1736.[12] He treated many famous patients, including Johann Sebastian Bach, Edward Gibbon,[13,14] and possibly George Frederick Handel.[15–17] In addition to the title "Chevalier," which he started

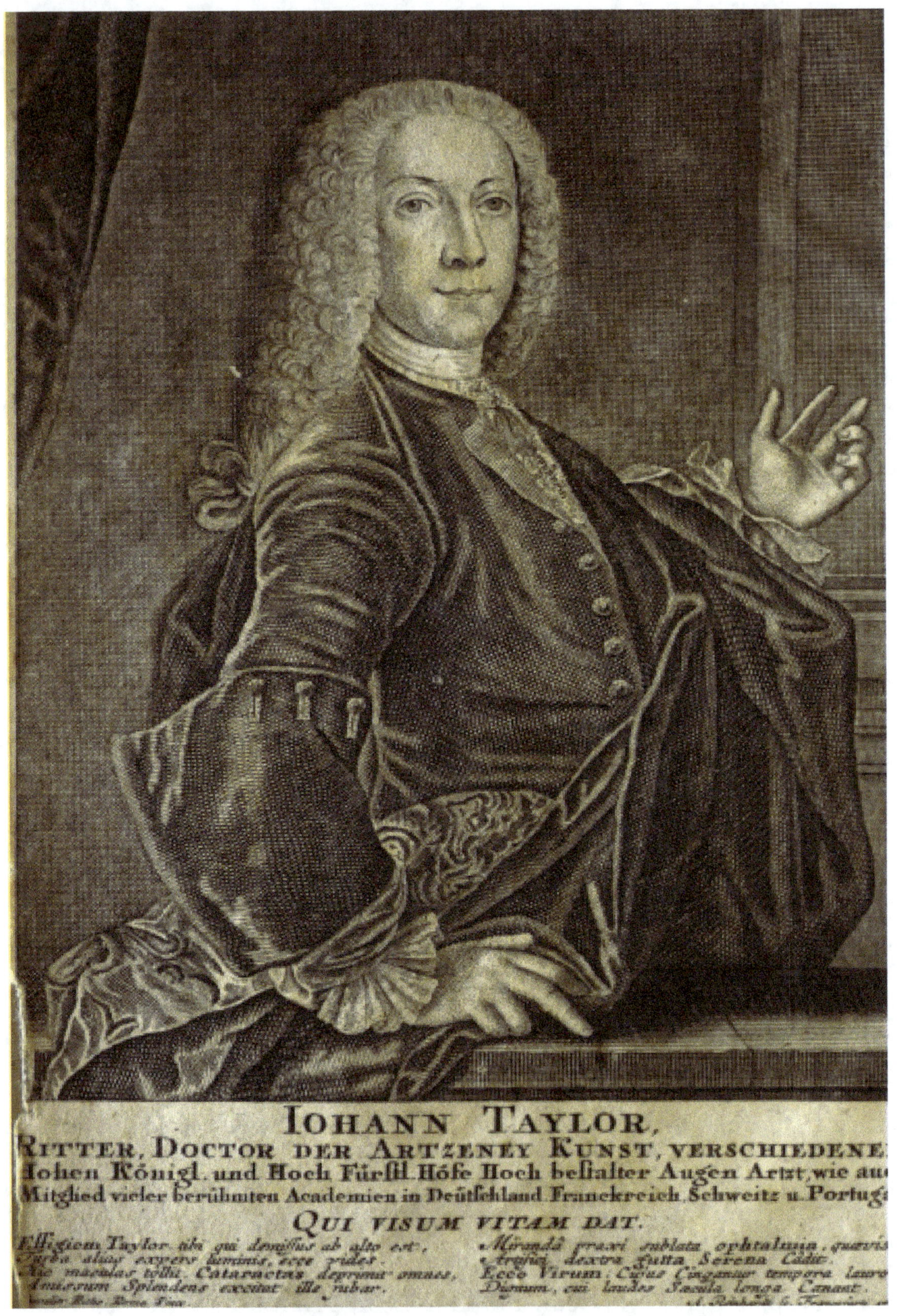

Fig. 1. Chevalier John Taylor.[24]

using consistently about 1750, he also named himself "Ophthalmiater Pontifical, Imperial and Royal."[18,19]

The precise details of his death are unknown. His grandson John wrote in 1832, "After many years absence from this country, my grandfather's death was noticed in the following manner in a continental paper: 'Having given sight to many thousands, the celebrated Chevalier Taylor lately died blind, at a very advanced age; in a convent at Prague'."[3] If the reports of Taylor's visual loss are true, they might help to explain why Taylor's surgical results, and reputation, appeared to worsen later in his life. For example, in 1768–1769, Taylor was reportedly forced by the Count Palatine in Mannheim to refund his surgical fees to many patients with unfavorable outcomes.[20] Similarly, in Prague in 1769, he was given the "consilium abeundi" (advice to leave) and was forbidden to perform eye surgery in the Habsburg territories.[21]

Taylor's many difficulties extended to his personal life. He seems to have insufficiently supported his wife, Ann (nee King), leading to tension between the Chevalier and his son John. The son wrote in 1761 that he had to financially support his mother.[22] A notice printed in 1759 does not name the Chevalier but appears to be targeting him: "Whereas a certain flaring itinerant Oculist, of England, now travelling about the Country has run from his Bail: This is to acquaint him, That if he does not make immediate Satisfaction to his Son, his Name will be publish'd, and a Reward for taking him. N.B. He also left his Wife in Distress, to whom he has been married between thirty and forty years."[23]

Taylor's care was criticized throughout his career, but his writings suggest a knowledge base at least as good as, and possibly much better than, those of his contemporaries.[24] For example, he wrote in 1735, "... there are no membranous Cataracts; but ... all Cataracts are from an Alteration of the chrystalline Humour itself."[25] This statement suggests a relatively "modern" understanding that a cataract is an opacity of the lens itself, rather than (as was classically thought) an opacity anterior to the lens. He also performed the relatively advanced procedure of optical iridotomy, which he described as creating an "artificial pupil."[26]

Taylor is credited with the first illustration of the semidecussation of the optic nerves through the chiasm in 1738, which he repeated in at least one other book (Fig. 2).[24,27–29] Taylor's description of what would now be described as phacomorphic glaucoma or pupillary block included: "... the Volume of the Chrystalline is so greatly augmented, as to raise the Circumference of the Pupil towards the Cornea, and violently press on the Uvea ... as to occasion ... a preternatural Pressure on the immediate Organ of Sight ..."[30]

Taylor claimed to have performed successful strabismus surgery,[31] although objective evidence of this has not been found. Nevertheless, his writings demonstrate a relatively advanced understanding of eye movement disorders[24,32] (Fig. 3). In 1766, Taylor published the *Nova Nosographia Ophthalmica* (New Description of Ophthalmic Diseases),[33] which is thought to be the first pictorial atlas of eye diseases, almost a century before that of Frédéric Jules Sichel.[34]

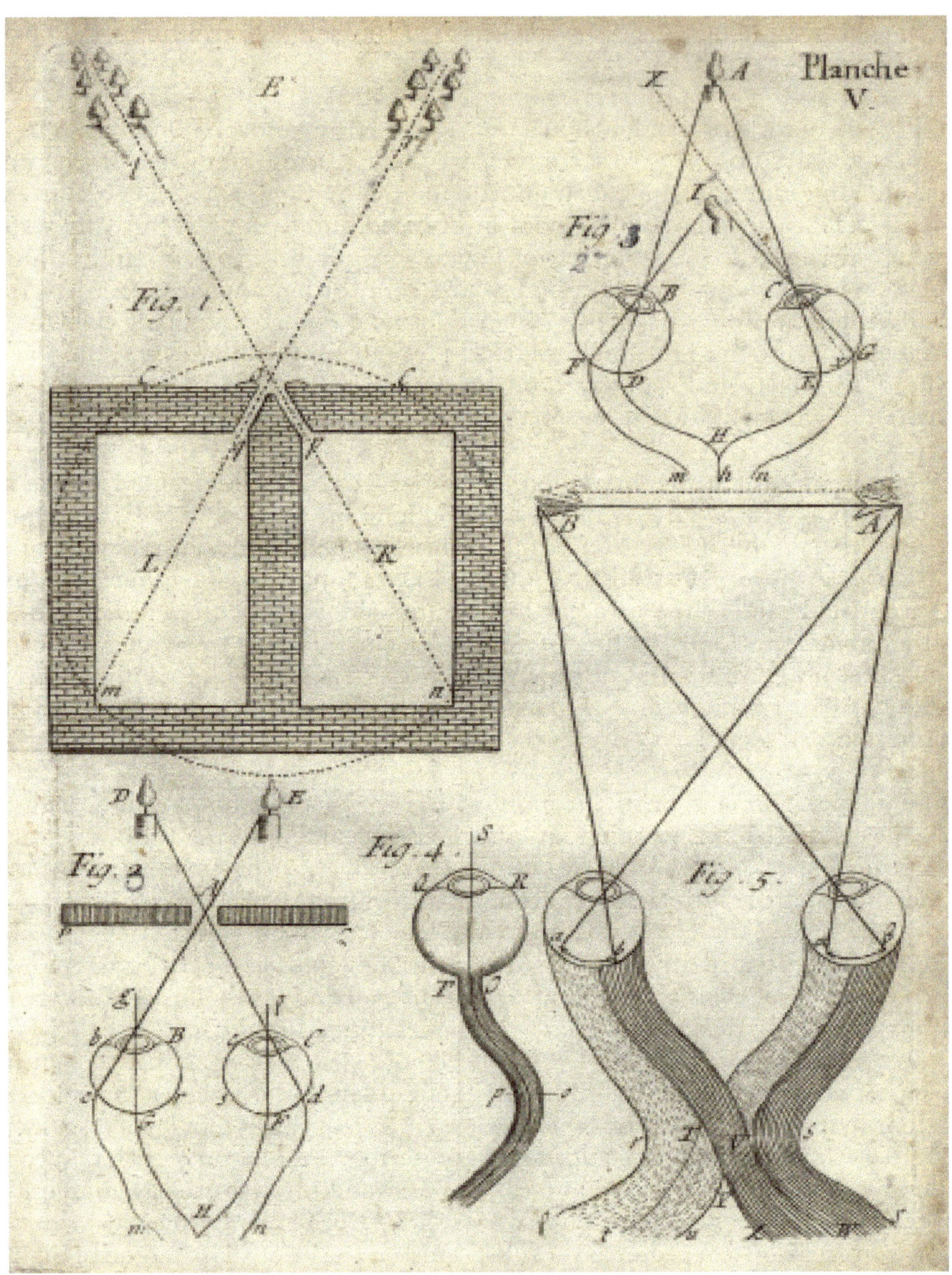

Fig. 2. Chevalier Taylor's illustration of the semidecussation of the optic nerves.[24]

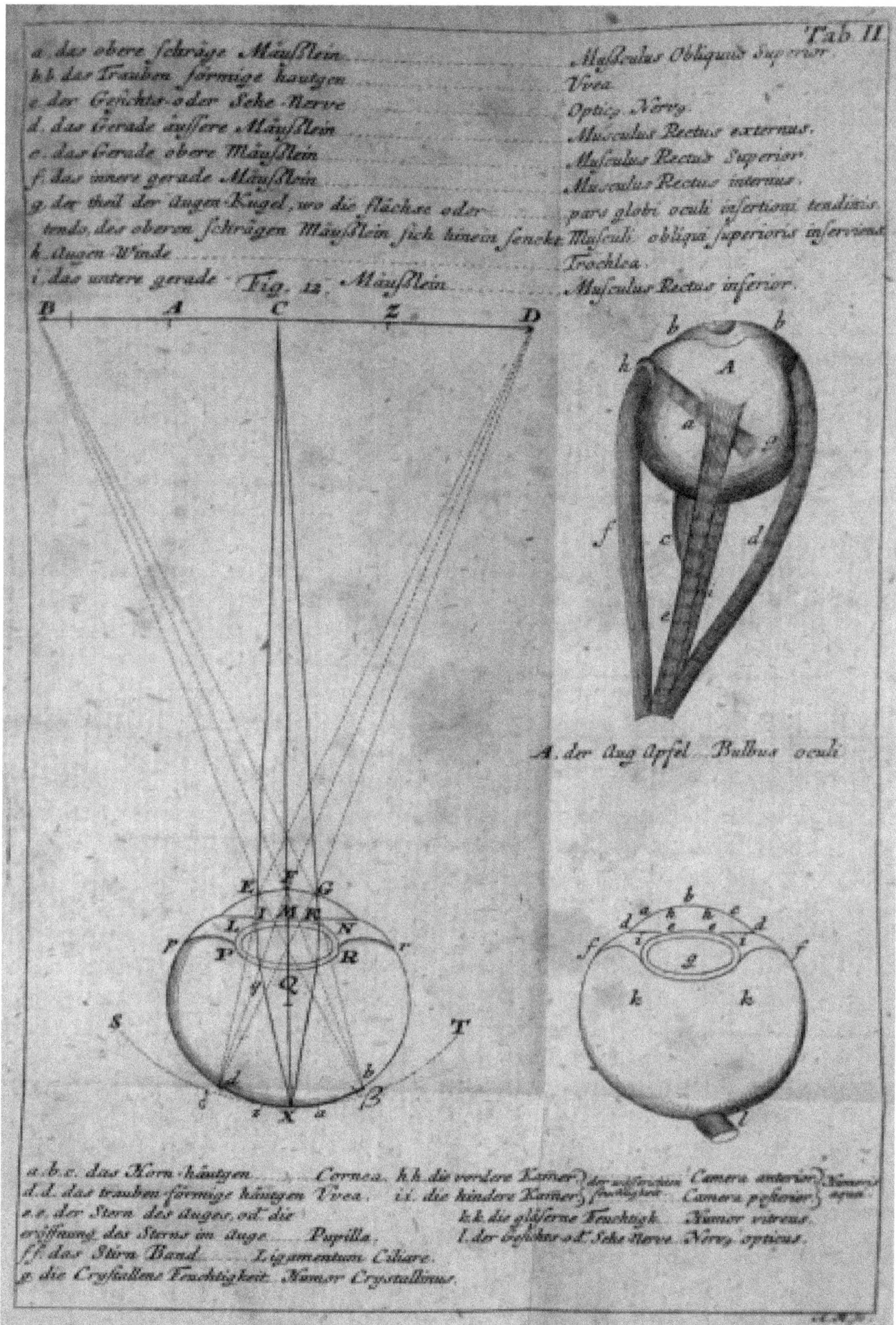

Fig. 3. Chevalier Taylor's diagram of the extraocular muscles, as well as other drawings.[24]

91

It is challenging, after more than two centuries, to evaluate Taylor's surgical outcomes. Taylor's descriptions of his techniques are self-aggrandizing and difficult to accept from a 21st-century perspective. Nevertheless, the journalist H. Cross-Grove wrote in 1742: "I was an Eye-Witness to his restoring to Sight Two Persons at my House on Thursday last ... which Two Persons in a few Minutes had so perfect a Sight, as to distinguish Objects ..."[35] A testimonial from 12 patients in 1742 reported, "Dr. JOHN TAYLOR, Oculist to the King, recovered our perfect Sight, after having intirely [sic] lost it many Years ..."[36]

Taylor famously operated on Bach in Leipzig in 1750, although the specific facts of the case are unknown. It has been suggested that Taylor performed couching, and the patient developed postoperative severe glaucoma,[16,37] although this has been disputed.[38,39] Following surgery, Bach was reported to have severe ocular pain, and he died several months later following a stroke. Taylor wrote: "... at *Leipsick*, where a celebrated master of music ... received his sight by my hands; it is with this very man that the famous *Handel* was first educated, and with whom I once thought to have had the same success, having all circumstances in his favour, motions of the pupil, light, &c. but upon drawing the curtain, we found the bottom defective, from a paralytic disorder."[11] Taylor's description suggests that the surgery (if it were couching) appeared to be successful, although the vision did not improve, perhaps due to pre-existing retinal or optic nerve disease.

Taylor was a controversial figure during his lifetime and mixed opinions about him persist. His contemporary Gerhard Ten Haaff (1720–1791) wrote of "de Beruchte [the infamous] TAYLOR" and his many surgical patients who became "geheel [completely] blind."[40] Samuel Johnson (1709–1784) mocked Taylor as an example of "how far impudence may carry ignorance,"[41] but Taylor's grandson John noted that the Chevalier's fluency in Latin was "a full refutation of the insolent abuse of my grandfather by Dr. Johnson."[3]

The Oxford professor William King (1685–1763) wrote of a relative, Sir William Smyth, who was successfully couched by Taylor ("Sir William was able to read and write without the use of spectacles during the rest of his life") but who then cheated Taylor out of most of his surgical fee by feigning visual loss.[42] King described Taylor: "He seems to have understood the anatomy of the eye perfectly well; he has a fine hand and good instruments, and performs all his operations with great dexterity; for the rest, *Ellum homo confidens!* [Look, there is a confident man!] who undertakes any thing (even impossible cases) and promises every thing. No charlatan ever appeared with fitter and more excellent talents, or to a greater advantage ..."[42]

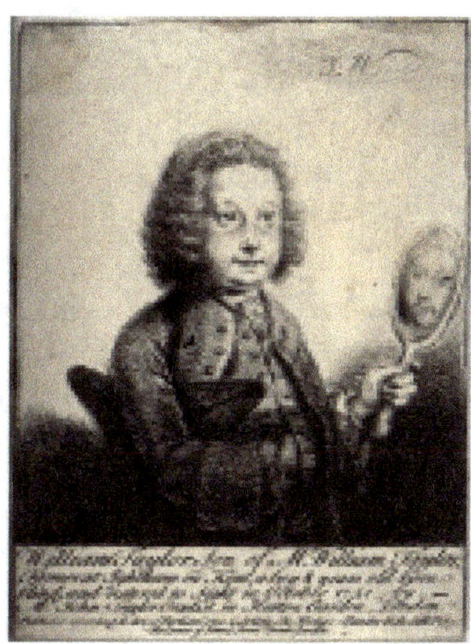

Fig. 4. The apparently unrelated 8-year-old William Taylor, whom John Taylor Jr. successfully operated for congenital cataracts.[44]

John Taylor, Jr. (1724–1787)

Taylor had one son, also named John,[17] who typically referred to himself as "John Taylor, Jr.," although he was at least the third consecutive John in the family. He was trained by his father, although he did not receive a medical degree. Although less flamboyant than his father, Taylor, Jr. appears to have been a very successful surgeon, who remained in London and provided much charity care. His own son (also named John), wrote that Taylor, Jr.'s "first great patient was the Duke of Ancaster ... the Duke had nearly succeeded in procuring for him the honour of being oculist to King George the Third, but the Duke of Bedford having had an operation for the cataract successfully performed by the Baron de Wenzel, obtained the appointment for the Baron."[3] Taylor, Jr. was reported to have successfully operated on at least two patients with congenital cataracts, including an apparently unrelated 8-year-old boy named William Taylor (Fig. 4).[43,44] Taylor Jr.'s friend William Oldys (1696–1761) wrote of the patient: "... he was set before a Looking-glass, and was greatly delighted with the little Man he saw in it, whom he would have to be his *own Man*, because he so obediently imitated, or repeated all the Motions and Gestures, which he made, with his Head, Mouth, and Hands; but said, *He would not close his Eyes* ..."[43] Congenital cataract surgery was considered especially challenging and was not reported in the English language until 1663.[45]

John Taylor, III (1757–1832)

Taylor, Jr. had 11 children. John, the Chevalier's grandson, was the first born.[3] He referred to himself as either "John Taylor" or "John Taylor, III," even though he was at least the fourth consecutive John in the family. Taylor, III had a less distinguished ophthalmic career than his father and grandfather, although he was appointed Oculist to the Prince of Wales in 1789.[46] Taylor, III and his younger brother Jeremiah (died 1822) were then appointed Oculists to King George III in 1790.[47,48] Taylor, III eventually quit ophthalmic practice to focus on a career as a writer and journalist. In 1795, his friend, the poet Robert Merry (1755–1798), following a professional misunderstanding, called Taylor, III "THE REPTILE OCULIST."[49] Some historians have confused Taylor, III with another John Taylor of approximately the same age, who was involved in several dramatic and public adventures in the early 1790s, including a serving as a government informant and a conviction for bigamy. It seems certain, however, that Taylor, III was not this latter John Taylor.[41]

Summary

Chevalier John Taylor was a colorful and controversial figure. Although his professional legacy is mixed, his personal legacy is much more favorable. Collectively, the lives of Taylor and his descendants illustrate ophthalmic practice in 18th- and 19th-century Europe.

Acknowledgement:

The authors of this chapter wish to acknowledge the assistance of Andrzej Grzybowski, Hans-Reinhard Koch, and Dennis Bermudez

References

1. Trevor-Roper P. Chevalier Taylor – Ophthalmiater Royal (1703-1772). Doc Ophthalmol. 1989;71:113–122.
2. Schwartz SG, Leffler CT, Grzybowski A, Koch H-R, Bermudez D. The Taylor dynasty: three generations of 18th-19th century oculists. Hist Ophthalmol Int. 2015;1:67–81.
3. Taylor J III. Records of My Life, Vol. 1. London: Edward Bull; 1832.
4. Taylor J. D'Avignon le 7. AoÛt ... Jeudi passé M. Taylor Oculiste Anglois arriva ... Les Professeurs & Docteurs en Medecine de nôtre Université ... l'ont aggregé dans leurs corps .... Courrier d'Avignon 64 (10. AoÛt); 1734:4.
5. Morénas F. Par ordre de mes Superieurs, je suis obligé de me retracter & de me dédire de ce que imprudemment & sur la sinple assertion du Sr. Taylor Oculiste Anglois, j'annoncai dans la Feüille precedente .... Courrier d'Avignon 65 (13. AoÛt); 1734:4.
6. Wood S. A rare manuscript of Chevalier Taylor, the Royal Oculist, with notes on his life. Br J Ophthalmol. 1930;14:193–223.
7. Taylor J. Lettre à MM. de l'Académie de Chirurgie sur l'art de rétablir la vue obscurcie par la maladie connue sous le nom de cataracte. Où l'on démontre les dangereuses conséquences de l'opération de la cataracte par extraction. Paris; 1766.
8. Figarella J. Jacques Daviel, maître chirurgien de Marseille, oculiste du Roi (1693-1763). Marseille: Jeanne Laffitt; 1979.

9. Koch H-R. Jacques Daviels Kampf um Anerkennung. (Annual Meeting of the Julius-Hirschberg-Gesellschadt in Köln, 2010). In F Krogmann (ed.). Mitteilungen der Julius-Hirschberg-Gesellschaft zur Geschichte der Augenheilkunde, Vol. 12. Würzburg: Königshausen & Neumann; 2014:117–175.

10. Blodi FC (trans.), Hirschberg J. The History of Ophthalmology, Vol. 3. The Renaissance of Ophthalmology in the Eighteenth Century (Part One). Bonn: J.P. Wayenborgh Verlag; 1984:152.

11. Taylor J. The History of the Travels and Adventures of the Chevalier John Taylor, Ophthalmiater; ... Written by Himself ... Addressed to His Only Son ... London; 1761–1762.

12. Lee S. Dictionary of National Biography, Vol. 55. New York: The Macmillan Company; 1898.

13. Gibbon E. Memoirs of His Life and Writings, Composed by Himself; Illustrated from His Letters, with Occasional Notes and Narrative, Published by John Lord Sheffield, Vol. 1. Dublin: P Wogan, L White et al.; 1796:19.

14. Jackson DM. Bach, Handel and the Chevalier Taylor. Med Hist. 1968;12:385–393.

15. Bäzner H, Hennerici MG. Georg Friedrich Händel's strokes. In: J Bogousslavsky, F Boller (eds.). Neurological Disorders in Famous Artists. Front Neurol Neurosci. 2005;19:150–159.

16. Tarkkanen A. Blindness of Johann Sebastian Bach. Acta Ophthalmol. 2013;91:191–192.

17. Coats G. The Chevalier Taylor. The Royal London Ophthalmic Hospital Reports. 1915;20:1–90.

18. Taylor J. Das merkwürdigste aus denen Wiener Relationen vom 3. Februarii ersiehet der Leser aus beygehendem Auszuge .... *Kurtz-gefaßte historische Nachrichten.* (6. Woche; February); 1751:115–116.

19. Taylor J. Wien. Freytag, den 6. dieses: Der Ritter Taylor Ihro Kaiserl. verwitweten Majestät zu Bayern ... ist hier angekommen – Le Chevalier Taylor Oculiste de S. M. Imp. l'Imperatrice douarriere de Baviere ... est arrivé ici .... *Wiener. Diarium* (89; 7 November); 1750:5.

20. Anon. De Manheim, le 3 May. Le Chevalier Taylor, Oculiste empirique, qui a soin de se faire annoncer d'avance dans les Villes, où il se propose d'opérer .... Nouvelles de Divers Endroits (Gazette de Berne) 40 (18. May, Suppl.); 1768:1–2.

21. Groß JH. Der renommierte Windbeutel, Chevallier Taylor, ist bey seinem letzten Creuzzug der Staar gut gestochen worden. Erlangische Real-Zeitung 54 (7. Juli); 1769:467.

22. Taylor J Jr. The Life and Extraordinary History of the Chevalier John Taylor, Member of the Most Celebrated Academies, Universities, and Societies of the Learned, ... Written from Authentic Materials, and Published by His Son, 2 Vols. London: M. Cooper; 1761.

23. Anon. Whereas a certain flaring itinerant Oculist ... London Evening Post (London, England), 6/9/1759–6/12/1759; Issue 4930; 1759.

24. Taylor J. Mechanismus oder Neue Abhandlung: von der künstlichen Zusammensezung des menschlichen Auges und den besondern Nuzen desselben, sowohl vor sich, als in Absicht der anliegenden Theile, nebst seiner Art, dessen Krankheiten zu heilen, Wie Ersolche bey einer mehr als zwanzigjährigen Erfahrung seiner durch Europa glüklich gethanen Augencuren bewährt befunden. Frankfurt am Mayn: Stocks seel. Erben und Schilling; 1750.

25. Anon. This Day is Published. General Evening Post (London, England), 12/20/1735–12/23/1735; Issue 348; 1735.

26. Mark HH. The strange report of Cheselden's iridotomy. Arch Ophthalmol. 2003;121:266–268.

27. Taylor J. Le méchanisme ou le nouveau traité de l'anatomie du globe de l'oeil, avec l'usage de ses différentes parties, & de celles qui lui sont contigués; orné de planches. Paris: Michel-Estienne David; 1738.

28. Rucker CW. The concept of a semidecussation of the optic nerves. AMA Arch Ophthalmol. 1958;59:159–171.

29. Wade NJ. Chevalier John Taylor, ophthalmiater. Perception. 2008;37:969–972.

30. Taylor J. A New Treatise on the Diseases of the Chrystalline Humour of a Human Eye: Or, of the Cataract and Glaucoma. London: James Roberts; 1736b:27–30.

31. Anon. We are desired to inform our Readers that Dr. Taylor, Occulist to his Majesty has at length found out a certain Method of removing that Defect called Squinting ... George Faulkner the Dublin Journal (Dublin, Ireland) 4/28/1747–5/2/1747; Issue 2100; 1747.

32. Berg F. The Chevalier Taylor and his strabismus operation. Br J Ophthalmol. 1967;51:667–673.

33. Taylor J. Nova nosographia ophthalmica; hoc est accurata receniso ducentorum et quadraginta trium affectuum, qui oculum humanum partesque vicinas ullo modo laedere aut ipsum visum adimere posssunt. Hamburg & Leipzig: Grund & HolleTaylor J Jr (1748): John Taylor, Oculist (Son of Dr. Taylor, Oculist to his Majesty), in Great Queen-Street, Linclon's-Inn-Fields... London Evening Post 3269 (October 13–15); 1766b:3.

34. Sichel FJ. Iconographie ophthalmologique ou description, avec figures coloriées, des maladies de l'organe de la vue, comprenant l'anatomie pathologique, la pathologie et la thérapeutique médico-chirurgicales, 2 Vols. Paris: J B Baillière et fils; 1852–1859.

35. Cross-Grove H. Cross-grove's news. Norwich Gazette (Norwich, England), 2/27/1742–3/6/1742; Issue 1848; 1742.

36. Good R, Vipond N, Beechino T, et al. Norwich, April 3. Norwich Gazette (Norwich, England), 3/27/1742–4/3/1742; Issue 1852; 1742.

37. Zegers RHC. The eyes of Johann Sebastian Bach. Arch Ophthalmol. 2005;123:1427–1430.

38. Ober WB. Bach, Handel and "Chevalier" John Taylor, MD: Ophthalmiater. N Y State J Med. 1969;69:1797–1807.

39. Grzybowski A. John Taylor and Johann Sebastian Bach – more information still needed. Acta Ophthalmol. 2013;91:250–252.

40. Ten Haaff G. Korte Verhandeling. Rotterdam: Reinier Arrenberg; 1761.

41. Barrell J. The reptile oculist. London Review of Books. 2004;26:19–25.

42. King W. Political and Literary Anecdotes of His Own Times. Boston: Wells and Lilly; 1819.

43. Oldys W. Observations on the Cure of William Taylor, the Blind Boy of Ightham, in Kent. Holborn, England: E. Owen; 1753.

44. Anon. This Day is publish'd, a Print of William Taylor, Son of William Taylor at Ightham in Kent ... and sold by Thomas Worlidge, Painter .... Daily Advertiser, Issue 6595 (February 26); 1752:2.

45. Leffler CT, Schwartz SG, Davenport B. Congenital cataract surgery during the early enlightenment period and the Stepkins oculists. JAMA Ophthalmol. 2014;132:883–884.

46. Anon. Carlton House, June 30. St. James's Chronicle or the British Evening Post (London, England), 7/7/1789–7/9/1789; Issue 4402; 1789.

47. Anon. Lord Chamberlain's Office, October 23. London Gazette (London, England), 10/19/1790–10/23/1790; Issue 13247; 1790.

48. Anon. Lord Chamberlain's Office, November 26, 1790. London Gazette (London, England), 11/23/1790–11/27/1790; Issue 13259; 1790.

49. Taylor J III. Records of My Life, Vol. 2. London: Edward Bull; 1832.

A *New History of Cataract Surgery* consists of:

* Chapters origination from: *The History of Ophthalmology – The Monographs 15: The History of Glaucoma*